Personal Growth and Development

GET A HANDLE ON ANXIETY

Calming Exercises for Anxiety and Panic Attacks

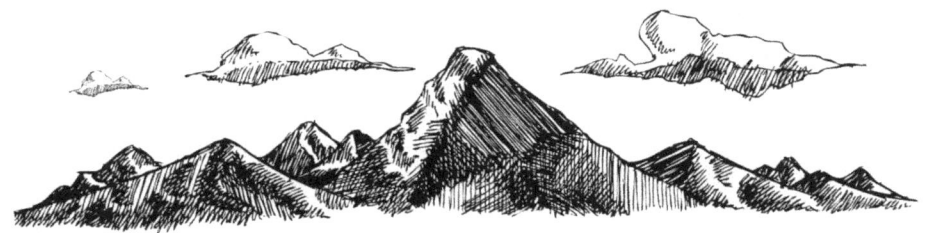

MONIQUE JOINER SIEDLAK

Oshun
Publications

Get a Handle on Anxiety © Copyright 2020 by Monique Joiner Siedlak

ISBN: 978-1-950378-41-8

All rights reserved

The content contained within this book may not be reproduced, duplicated or transmitted without direct written permission from the author or the publisher.

Under no circumstances will any blame or legal responsibility be held against the publisher, or author, for any damages, reparation, or monetary loss due to the information contained within this book, either directly or indirectly.

Legal Notice

This book is copyright protected. It is only for personal use. You cannot amend, distribute, sell, use, quote or paraphrase any part, or the content within this book, without the consent of the author or publisher.

Disclaimer Notice

Please note the information contained within this document is for educational and entertainment purposes only. All effort has been executed to present accurate, up to date, reliable, complete information. No warranties of any kind are declared or implied. Readers acknowledge that the author is not engaged in the rendering of legal, financial, medical or professional advice. The content within this book has been derived from various sources. Please consult a licensed professional before attempting any techniques outlined in this book.

By reading this document, the reader agrees that under no circumstances is the author responsible for any losses, direct or indirect, that are incurred as a result of the use of the information contained within this document, including, but not limited to, errors, omissions, or inaccuracies.

Cover Design by MJS

Cover Image by gunnar3000@ depositphotos.com

Published by Oshun Publications

www.oshunpublications.com

Contents

Other Books in Series	v
A Great Offer	vii
Introduction	xi
1. Is Anxiety Running Your Life?	1
2. Your Emotions	13
3. Your Body and Physical Sensations	17
4. Avoidance and Escape	19
5. Acceptance and Approach	21
6. What to Tell Yourself to Overcome Anxiety and Panic Attacks	27
7. Pushing Anxiety Over the Edge	35
8. How to Feel Safe Wherever You Are	43
9. How to Deal With a Fear of Failure	45
10. A Special on Panic Attacks	57
11. Exercises	63
12. Thought Versus Reality	75
13. Getting Unstuck From a Thought	79
14. The Road Ahead	81
Conclusion	85
References	87
About the Author	91
More Books by Monique Joiner Siedlak	93
Thank You!	95

Other Books in Series

Personal and Self Development
Creative Visualization
Astral Projection for Beginners
Meditation for Beginners
Reiki for Beginners
Manifesting With the Law of Attraction
Stress Management
Time Bound
Healing Animals with Reiki
Being an Empath Today

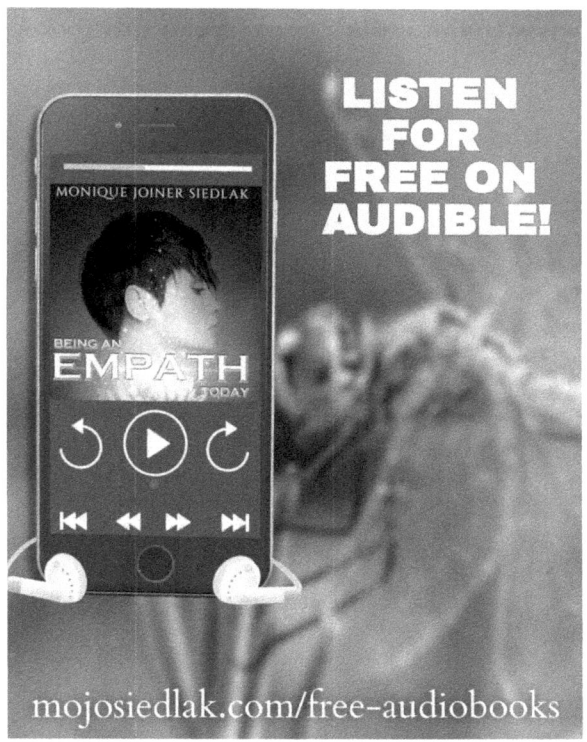

Want to learn about African Magic, Wicca, or even Reiki while cleaning your home, exercising, or driving to work? I know it's tough these days to simply find the time to relax and curl up with a good book. This is why I'm delighted to share that I have books available in audiobook format.

Best of all, you can get the audiobook version of this book or any other book by me for free as part of a 30-day Audible trial.

Members get free audiobooks every month and exclusive discounts. It's an excellent way to explore and determine if audiobook learning works for you.

If you're not satisfied, you can cancel anytime within the trial period. You won't be charged, and you can still keep your book. To choose your free audiobook, visit:

www.mojosiedlak.com/free-audiobooks

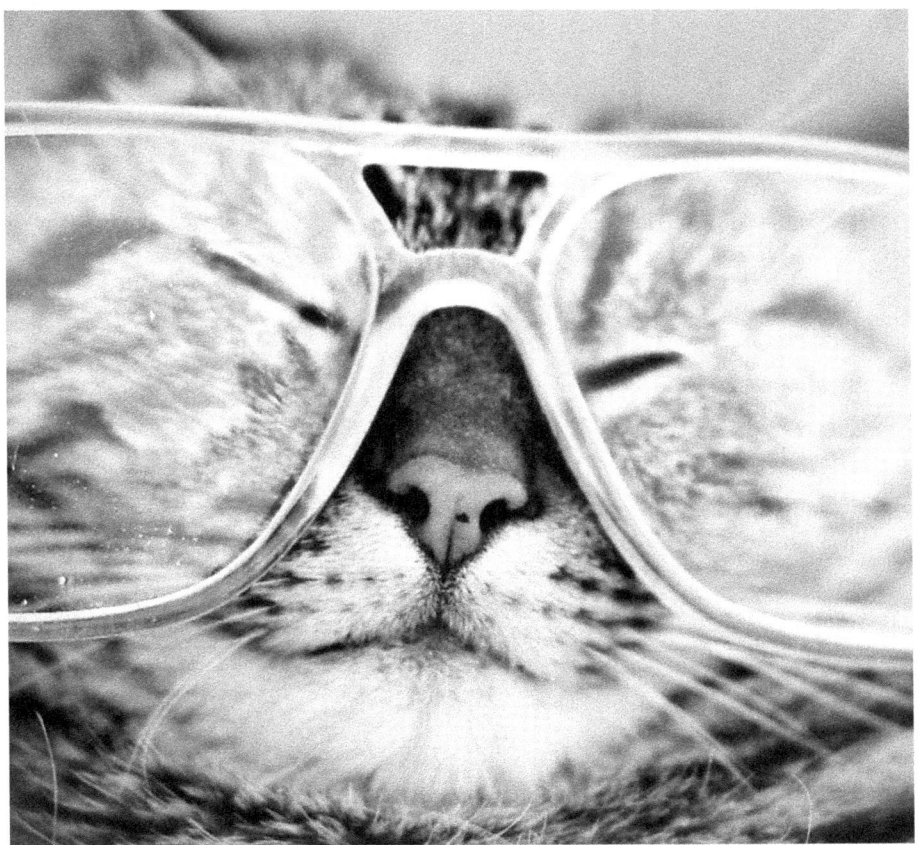

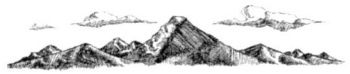

Introduction

Timon: "Hakuna Matata. What a wonderful phrase."

Pumba: "Hakuna Matata. Ain't no passing craze."

Timon: "It means no worries for the rest of your days."

Timon and Pumba: "It's a problem-free philosophy… Hakuna Ma…"

Timon: "…ma, wait! Pumba, I just gotta check my emails first. And my texts. And I haven't spoken to Simba and Lana and the new cubs in ages. And we need to get to the waterhole first before we hit the Antelope traffic! And… and I can't breathe, Pumba!"

Pumba: "Timon. Timon. I can't breathe either. I'm sweating like a hog. Even more than a hog. Why do I sweat more than other hogs? Aaahhh!"

Ah, just imagine this Disney classic if it were set in the 21st Century (and if these little critters had human brains, of course). It would seem like Hakuna Matata just wouldn't be the same as it was in the movie. Why?

If Timon and Pumba were to live like humans today, they'd probably be wrapped up in anxiety. Because of their primitive brains that would be so confused by all the stresses they would face today. In their natural, primitive surroundings, they would literally just fight, flee, or freeze if some predator or threat rocked up.

But if these characters were to live in our modern society today, there would be no primitive threats in a form they would recognize. They wouldn't have to rummage through the jungle for little bugs to eat – they could just safely pop into the next convenience store. Pumba would probably be an obese hog due to emotional overeating. Timon would probably be deeply insecure due to some popularity contest with other social media influencers. Who knows?

What I'm attempting to get at is though this whole scenario is not a reality, for most people today, anxiety is a reality. A big distorted reality.

In this book, we take a more in-depth look at the distorted reality that anxiety causes. We explore what anxiety means and determine whether your life is being run by this contagious emotion. We also explore in the simplest of ways, with simple language and simple solutions, this emotion that has become quite a complex phenomenon.

If we pick up some tell-tale signs that your Hakuna Matata is warped, we will pick you out with some great understanding and tools to manage this emotion that is so prominent in today's society. This way, you can get a grip on your anxiety and write your own version of a "problem-free philosophy" for life. So, are you ready to join me and reclaim the 'Tata' to your 'Hakuna'?

ONE

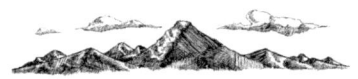

Is Anxiety Running Your Life?

We're going to determine whether anxiety is running your life or not. But before we can determine this, we need to be on the same page about what anxiety actually is and what it means.

So let's swing by the trusty Merriam-Webster dictionary. Ol' Merriam basically narrows the definition of anxiety down to:

1. An uncertain uneasiness or nervousness usually over an impending or anticipated ill. It is a state of being anxious.
2. A strange and overpowering sense of foreboding and fear generally marked by physical signs such as tension, sweat, and raised pulse rate, by uncertainty dealing with the reality and nature of the threat, and by self-doubt about one's strength to cope with it.
3. Mentally distressing concern or interest.
4. An intense desire frequently incorporated with doubt, fear, or uneasiness (Merriam-Webster, n.d.).

Boy, what a mouth full. Yet, still, I find a word missing in these descriptions of the name. The American Psychological Association (APA) mentions the word I'm looking for in their definition of anxiety:

Anxiety is an emotion (now that's what I'm talking about) identified by feelings of tension, troubling thoughts, and physical changes like raised blood pressure (APA, n.d.).

So though there are so many ways one can define anxiety, the essence of the word lies in the fact that it is a universal human emotion. We'll get a little deeper into your feelings in Chapter 2. For now, I'd like you to connect to the idea that anxiety is an emotion and not necessarily an illness.

I specifically mention that anxiety is not necessarily an illness. It is when our anxiety spins out of control that it can take over our lives and become truly toxic. If left unattended, anxiety could lead to phobias, panic attacks, depression, dread, chronic fatigue, etc. These could all be considered illnesses or just make you downright feel ill.

Before we get too deep into the pathology of anxiety, let's just take a quick look at the neuroscience behind anxiety. This is important because of how our brains and the mind-body connection functions is a crucial starting point in your journey of "getting a grip." We've already determined that anxiety is an emotion. An emotion that is mostly linked to some sort of fear or worry about the future. So let's just have a quick look at the relationship between fear and anxiety. This will lead us to some significant perspectives regarding the neuroscience of anxiety.

So, What's the Difference Between Fear and Anxiety?

Professor of neuroscience and director of the Emotional Brain Institute, Joseph LeDoux, gives a clear and simple distinction between fear and anxiety on BBC World Wide's The Forum podcast (2016).

LeDoux describes fear as a negative emotion that occurs when a threat is immediately present or likely to happen very shortly.

Whereas anxiety is a worried emotion about a future threat that may or may not happen. There is always an element of uncertainty when it comes to anxiety because the future is not a hundred percent certain.

What Relevance Do Fear and Anxiety Have in the Field of Neuroscience?

The amygdala. Ah, the infamous little almond-shaped mass in our limbic system shapes the way we perceive certain emotions - one of which is fear. This little minion in our brain stores memories of events and emotions we experienced to recognize similar events in the future... See what I'm getting at?

It is commonly believed that the amygdala might just be the root of our anxiety. Because of how the amygdala sends out impulses in reaction to what our brains experience as fear. And remember our distinction between fear and anxiety? Our amygdala tends to send an immediate response of fear when we experience a threat. Though fear is immediate when a threat is near, keep in mind that this little instinctive-emotional-almond has been storing past experiences of fear that are supposed to help us recognize similar situations in the future. And this is where anxiety starts to peek through.

Now before I continue, let's go over a brief breakdown of the three primary brain regions. The lower brain is pleased when we feel physically good. The limbic system is content when we are emotionally well. The higher brain (also known as the cortex) is fulfilled when we make good and healthy decisions for ourselves. The human brain is a wondrous thing, but one of the truly magical things is that these three brain regions have separate functions. Still, all three of them can merge and cooperate.

With this ebb and flow between the brain regions in mind, let's retake a look at the amygdala. Though this tiny part of the brain also processes other emotions, it has been strongly related to fear. Even to the extent that it earned itself the nickname the "seed of fear." In the same BBC World Wide's The Forum podcast (2016) I referred to earlier, Professor LeDoux argues that this actually has a misleading aspect to it. The more we dig into these things in the brain, the more we find that the processes that seem to be unified in our conscious minds are separate. He emphasizes that what is separate is the brain's ability to detect and respond to danger, as opposed to the ability to consciously experience fear or anxiety.

We aren't born with fear, nor are we hard-wired to fear. We learn to fear. We are conditioned to fear. As we move through life, we construct the experience of fear in our own mind and brain as the experience unfolds. What is wired into our brain are the processes of detecting or responding to fear. And once these processes are triggered - holy moly - there is a lot of stuff going on in terms of brain arousal and feedback from bodily responses. You have all of this physiological mojo going around that indirectly contributes to fear and anxiety. Still, it's not the same thing as the experience of fear and anxiety. This distinction is important because it affects the way therapies are developed in terms of drugs or psychotherapy.

Threat Reaction vs. Fear

So, you're out on a hike at a majestic outdoor location when suddenly you come to a halt: scorpion!

Your brain has detected the threat of the scorpion. You are frozen. But as you become *aware* of what is going on, you experience fear. Fear is the awareness that you are in danger.

In contrast, the brain's ability to detect and respond to danger is something entirely different.

This is an excellent example of where the interaction between the three brain regions comes into play again.

The lower brain is disrupted. It has gone from a state of being pleased with feeling satisfied because you were feeling physically good while walking in nature, to a state where your body starts reacting to the threat detected by the limbic system.

The limbic system is triggered by the detection of a threat. Hence you are not emotionally content anymore. Your fight, flight, or freeze response kicks in. The amygdala starts processing emotions arising from this trigger: fear, anxiety, overwhelmedness, surprise, etc. The lower brain picks up on all these emotional interpretations of the amygdala. It physically reacts through things like sweaty palms, shallow breathing, and increased heart rate.

While the chatter between the limbic system and the lower brain is ongoing, the higher brain comes into play. The higher brain, or cortex, is the perceiving and thinking part of the brain. This is where we can consciously choose and manage the triggered impulses and how we respond to it. It is also the part of your brain that allows you to read and understand what is written here. Through our higher brain, we can communicate to the limbic system that the threat is not real or not immense. And if we calm the limbic system, the lower brain acts accordingly in managing its physical responses. The vice versa is also true. The higher brain can consciously engage with the lower brain and calm the physical reactions and processes in the body. This can also settle the emotional responses in the lower brain. How amazing is that?

Now back to the scorpion that set off this brainy trio's interaction:

Lower Brain: "Yikes! Scorpion. Freeze!"

Limbic System: "Wait, what? Oh crap. I'm scared."

Lower Brain: "You're afraid? Oh no. We need more oxygen, guys. Lungs! Pick up your breathing pace! Heart, you better put your foot on the accelerator and pick up the pace - we need blood rushing! This is not a drill! I repeat this is not a drill! The limbic system reports a real threat!"

Higher Brain: "All right, you two, papa's here. I checked it out. It's not a scorpion. It's actually a piece of bark. But don't feel embarrassed Limbic System, it's okay. Rather safe than sorry. It could have been a scorpion - I know you're sensitive to them because you were stung as a kid. But the three of us are alright. Hey, Lower Brain, you can tell the rest of the body to chill now. Thanks."

See, on the surface, that whole reaction is generally perceived as a crazy "all-in-one" reaction. But it's really not. In this example, I actually used a kind of "ideal conversation" or intervention by conscious higher brain activity. However, this is generally not the case. And it is especially not the case when it comes to anxiety. It all depends on how we've been conditioned to act on specific triggers or responses.

But can you see that I'm planting a seed of hope here? If you can create an awareness in your higher brain, to manage what's going on between the lower mind and your limbic system, anxiety and the emotional and physical elements connected to it can be achieved.

What the higher brain was getting at in its conversation was that it's not all bad to mistake a piece of bark for a scorpion. However, if this "mistake" keeps repeating and prevents you from wanting to ever walk in nature again… well then, Houston, we have a problem. Then, my dear friend, anxiety might just be running your life.

Make sense?

The Anxiety Disorder Spectrum as a Means to Determine if Anxiety Is Running Your Life

Because anxiety is an emotion that comes down to worry about the future, it's been called the "price tag on our freedom" by some. One might also say that it's the price we pay for having a brain that can anticipate the future. Just like in the example of the piece of bark being mistaken for a scorpion. If we could not predict the future, there would be a much lower level of anxiety going about.

All you have to let "settle in" is that when our anticipation of the future becomes much more weighted than our engagement in the present, you probably have a good chance of anxiety sticking out its head.

This does, however, beg the question: to what extent is anxiety welcome in my life?

At this point, it would be good to have a chat about the anxiety disorder spectrum. See, fear is an emotion that is actually geared to protect us, but it can be harmful if we have too much fear or start functioning from a place of fear. It is then that fear begins to rule our lives. In such a case, fear is not protecting us anymore; it's inhibiting us and making our lives small.

The same goes for anxiety. Anxiety isn't all bad. It lies on a spectrum that, on one end, can surface as low levels of fear or apprehension. Subtle sensations of muscle stiffness, sweating, or something as simple as doubting the ability you have to complete a particular task. It is important to note that typical symptoms of anxiety will not interfere with your daily functioning. A little anxiety may actually assist in motivating you to work harder towards your goals or warn you about potential threats alongside your intuition.

For example, if you have a big presentation coming up at work, anxiety about the task may drive you to thoroughly prepare for the task. Or anxiety experienced by a pedestrian might just allow them to get out of the way of a speeding car which they weren't aware of. These examples show how normal levels of anxiety can be of good use in everyday life.

However, on the other end of the spectrum, one finds clinical levels of anxiety in the form of diagnosable disorders. These disorders occur when your levels of anxiety increase so drastically that your performance and daily functioning decreases or becomes impaired.

In the middle of the spectrum, there is a kind of "grey zone." This middle ground is referred to as the "almost anxious" area of the anxiety disorder spectrum by many therapists. In this zone, your level of anxiety edges on a negative impact on your life. Here, anxiety isn't conducive to productivity anymore. It is neither helpful nor adaptive to performance, and it starts to erect a barrier to a joyful life. However, it doesn't really yet meet the diagnostics of an anxiety disorder - you are just "almost anxious." You may find yourself consumed by negative thoughts and fear, which creates a struggle to focus on your tasks at hand.

If someone is "almost anxious," they might find themselves procrastinating at their desks all day. Worrying about things instead of just working on the task in front of them. They might experience physical sensations like the tightness of muscles or a clenched feeling in their stomach. I'm not talking stiffness due to crunches that build abs here people. I'm talking on-the-edge-of-a-stomach-ulcer… Aaah. In such a case, anxiety hasn't surfaced to the extent that it prevented the person from showing up for work. Still, it did inhibit their ability to function at work.

The "almost-anxious" grey zone is a great place to start paying attention to your anxiety levels. If you do not get a grip on your anxiety, anxiety will get a hold on you! Consequently, before you know it, anxiety can consume your life and tip you over into the clinical side of the anxiety disorder spectrum.

Just so we're clear: in this book, we will mostly speak to the lower and middle end of the anxiety disorder spectrum. Though the tools in this book will most definitely help cope with a clinical anxiety disorder, the best thing would still be to seek professional help. And when you do seek help, take care to find out if the psychiatrist you are consulting is trained in the amygdala. As well as cortex-based strategies for reducing anxiety such as cognitive behavioral therapy. People sometimes confuse psychiatrists with therapists - don't step into that judgment error. Psychiatrists are trained physicians that treat psychological disorders, primarily through medication. A psychiatrist might even recommend a therapist in conjunction with medication. But a psychiatrist that is not trained in cognitive behavioral therapy might have a substantial focus on the use of drugs. Where anxiety is very much related to the mind-body connection and how the brain works. So you should be a little picky in this sense.

Now that we understand which parts of our brains are primarily responsible for our emotional and physical well-being, and where our power and consciousness lies, we'll take a more in-depth look into our emotions in Chapter 2. Followed by a talk about our bodies and the physical sensations linked to anxiety in Chapter 3. If you are still unclear as to where you lie on the anxiety spectrum, here are some questions to guide you in determining your position.

Self-Assessment Exercise: Where Do I Rank on the Anxiety Disorder Spectrum?

To find out, complete the self-assessment questions below, answering "mostly yes" or "mostly no" to each question.

- Do you have trouble falling or staying asleep?
- Do you find it hard to relax?
- Do you sometimes feel fearful for no reason?
- Do you often find yourself with a dry mouth?

- Do you often feel overwhelmed?
- Are you only as happy as the people around you?
- Are you afraid of crowds, being left alone, the dark, of strangers or of traffic?
- Do you often have nightmares?
- Do you find yourself thinking a lot about why you do the things you do?
- Are you a worrier?
- Do you avoid social gatherings or situations because of nervousness, fear, or anxiety?
- Are you very concerned about what people think of you?
- Do you feel that you never laugh enough?
- Do you often feel tired and lack energy?
- Do you find yourself always busy but not productive?
- Do you sit and think about a problem for hours and then still feel like it has not been resolved?
- Do you have frequent headaches or neck pain?
- Do you find yourself having less interest in activities that you usually find joy in?
- Do you often feel like you are losing control over everything in your life?
- Are you afraid that you might find yourself in a situation where you are unable to escape in a hurry?

Now let's calculate your results:

If you answered yes to one to five questions, you're most likely dealing with general, day-to-day anxiety and can efficiently utilize your anxiety in your favor. You need to motivate yourself and identify potential threats before they cause harm.

If you answered yes to six to fourteen questions, you're in the "almost-anxious" grey zone. Your anxiety is not running your life completely. Still, it does have more of a grip on you than you on it. Your anxiety is not conducive to your productivity levels. It is likely erecting a barrier that makes it hard for you to live a joyful life.

If you answered yes to more than fifteen questions, it looks like anxiety is running your life in an all-consuming capacity. It might be good to seek professional help if you feel like your anxiety is impairing your ability to lead a normal happy life.

Oh here is a little disclaimer: this questionnaire is by no mean a diagnosis. It is just an indication of the route you might want to follow to live your best life! If you strongly believe you have a deeper underlying issue relating to anxiety, seek professional help from a psychologist or psychiatrist. As for the rest, I can't wait to continue this journey to finding your Hakuna-Matata-mojo!

TWO

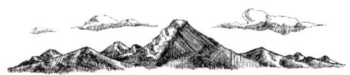

Your Emotions

IN THE PREVIOUS CHAPTER, WE TOOK A LOOK AT THE THREE brain regions and their primary functions. It is vital to have a background of knowledge as to how our brains operate. It gives us a wealth of insight into how we can understand anxiety and how we can engage with and manage it.

When it comes to our emotions, the limbic system comes into play as it is responsible for our emotional well-being. We touched on the role of the little almond-shaped amygdala in the limbic system. Still, here we'll take a more in-depth look into its function and how it relates to our emotions and anxiety in particular.

A Look Into Nature

So the amygdala is mainly responsible for detecting and responding to danger. It is also accountable for how we interpret our experiences of the danger we recognize through emotions like fear, anxiety, anger, and sadness.

Let's look to nature to better understand the amygdala and how our human brains might engage and react differently from other animal species when it comes to fear and anxiety.

All vertebrates, including birds, fish, amphibians, reptiles, and mammals, have an amygdala. And in these cases, its primary function is to detect and respond to threats. However, the ability to experience fear or anxiety only occurs in a brain capable of being conscious of its own activities. That's why the human brain is so special. Humans are the only species we know of for sure that has a brain capable of being conscious.

This doesn't mean that other animals don't have some kind of conscious experience, but I mean scientifically speaking, we don't really have a way of going into an animal's brain and verifying that this capability exists.

From this point of view, we can study threat processing and detection in humans and animals. Still, the conscious study of fear and anxiety, we need to do in humans.

The average person can usually only verbalize up to three emotions due to a lack of emotional vocabulary. People tend to be able to voice that they are sad, happy, or angry. Obviously, there are more, but we're working on the worst-case scenario here.

When we can better express our emotions, we can feel that we have a grip on them. We can acknowledge them and explore where they come from, what triggered them, and then take it from there.

Ironically, we don't usually express that we feel anxious because, for some reason, there is a stigma connected to anxiety. Yet anxiety is one of the most contagious emotions, if not the most infectious, from my perspective.

Researcher-Storyteller, Dr. Brené Brown, compiled a list of core emotions most people experience, but don't necessarily have the emotional vocabulary to express.

Brené Brown List of Core Emotions

Anger	Disgust	Gratitude	Jealous	Regret
Anxious	Embarrassed	Grief	Joy	Sad
Belonging	Empathy	Guilt	Judgment	Shame
Blame	Excited	Happy	Lonely	Surprised
Curious	Fear/Scared	Humiliation	Love	Vulnerability
Disappointed	Frustrated	Hurt	Overwhelmed	Worried

Now that we have some sexy, emotional vocabulary in our back pockets, let's run through the stages of emotions. By nature, emotions are quite volatile and irrational. Why do we have to feel happy or sad? Why do we even have emotions at all? My point is that we'll probably never be able to fully understand them. But since we can at least name and know them, we can try and understand why they show up. We can learn what they want to show us.

Anxiety and Its Relationship to Other Emotions

Though anxiety is an emotion in its own right, it has a family. And it's a complicated family. Because when anxiety participates, it tends to drag all the naughty negative cousins along. And the issues surrounding anxiety get the negative-emotion-cousins all shook up. Scenarios such as anxiety attacks, experiencing anxiety in front of someone close to you, or feeling like you're the only person in the world dealing with anxiety can all evoke strings of other anxiety-related emotions like loneliness, shame, frustration, sadness, etc.

All of these emotions are caused by anxiety in a sense, but they can all lead to other emotional issues too. If you do not develop the coping skills to manage your anxiety, other emotions might spiral out of control. Each of the negative emotions harnessed by anxiety brings issues that need resolution in their own right. Hence, anxiety can cause some negative feelings, and some negative emotions can create anxiety. So it's important to check in with your emotions and ask where they are coming from and what they are trying to communicate to you.

THREE

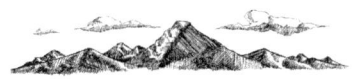

Your Body and Physical Sensations

ANXIETY ISN'T ONLY IN OUR MINDS. IT HAS A POWERFUL physical sensation that manifests in the body. The extent to which it surfaces, on a very tangible physical level, depends strongly on the level of anxiety that a person is experiencing.

The anxiety that is left unattended runs the risk of escalating and eventually turns into an anxiety disorder. This can interfere with your life and almost suck out all joy from your existence. No joke. Types of anxiety orders you might have heard of include panic disorders, separation anxiety, social anxiety, generalized anxiety disorder, phobias, and obsessive-compulsive behavior (OCD).

The physical symptoms you can experience when any of these disorders strike or experience a significant level of anxiety may include:

- Stomach upsets like nausea, cramps, or digestive issues.
- Headaches.
- Sleeplessness or general trouble with falling and staying asleep.
- Chronic fatigue.

- A feeling of physical weakness.
- A rapid heart rate or a very prominent pounding heart.
- Sweating.
- Trembling and shaking.
- Muscle tension, spasms, or pain.

These are general bodily sensations caused by anxiety. Still, certain anxiety disorders, such as panic disorders, may have even more extreme physical symptoms. But we'll have a more thorough look at that in chapter 5.

We already know that anxiety is mostly our body's emotional reaction to a detected danger or threat. This reaction we also call our fight, flee, or freeze (FFF-reaction) reaction. The tricky thing is, our bodies aren't made to function optimally in a vigilant state all the time. If you reside in a constant FFF-reaction state, it could have severe repercussions for your physical health.

Tensed muscles, for example, can naturally prepare you to rush out of a danger zone. Still, if these muscles stay tense all the time, it can result in a lot of pain, such as migraines and tension headaches.

We have two hormones, adrenaline and cortisol, that increase our heart rate and breathing to face a threat. However, these hormones also affect your digestion and blood sugar levels. So if you are stressed and anxious over an extended period, the frequent release of these hormones can affect your health, including how your body's digestive system functions. Some studies showed that anxiety symptoms have been linked with ulcers, vision problems, back problems, heart problems, and even asthma.

So if you are experiencing high levels of stress and anxiety, it's vitally important that you get a grip on it. It hinders your well-being on an emotional level. Still, it can have devastating effects on your body in the long-term.

FOUR

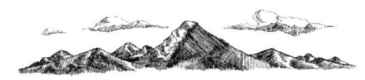

Avoidance and Escape
_____

OKAY, I'M GOING TO LET YOU IN ON A LITTLE SECRET. Contrary to popular belief, sometimes the best thing you can do to calm your anxiety is to just let it happen. Just sit with it. Don't avoid it. Don't escape it. Just allow it. Sounds kind of counterintuitive, doesn't it?

You see, when we minimize or catastrophize our anxiety, we kind of invalidate it. The thing is, anxiety is a healthy, valid emotion, and we should deal with it accordingly.

Most people seem to think that we need to stay busy and productive, so we don't have time to sit and ponder upon all the anxious thoughts we have inside. Here's where it gets tricky, though. Quite often, these buzzing environments can ignite your anxiety. This happens because you are aware that you feel anxious, so you just stay busy in an environment that is demanding you to be productive. This can lead to a form of "imposter syndrome" where you feel like a fraud because actually you're just being busy but not really producing anything of worth.

The same goes for avoiding anxiety-provoking scenarios. It's also some form of procrastination. And if you really think about it, procrastination is really just telling you that you are anxious or stressed about a situation. When we avoid things, we are choosing the path of least resistance.

The truth is, we really need to learn to live in balance with anxiety. Just like we live with any other emotions. Anxiety is a universal human emotion. Every single person experiences anxiety to some extent. Anxiety is a natural response to specific encounters. If we keep on ignoring it or shoving it out of the way, it will just crawl more profound and deeper into our insides.

At its best, anxiety can help us keep us focused and alert by getting our hearts pounding and releasing extra adrenaline into our bodies. But it can also wreak havoc and impair our vigor and abilities to the point of inaction.

Can you think of any examples of how anxiety and avoidance have interfered with your day-to-day life? It might be helpful to jot them down in a journal. Now envision the goals you want to reach and identify the ones that anxiety might prevent you from reaching. Be sure you take a good look at the future and beyond your daily life. Is anxiety giving you an excuse to avoid specific action steps in your life? Is it preventing you from taking that trip to Thailand or ditching the job you're loathing or telling someone that you like them?

If so, stop avoiding the uncomfortable zones in your life where anxiety is slowing you down. Accept that you have anxiety in your life, but also accept the responsibility of managing it! In our next chapter, we'll be sharing some valuable tools and strategies to navigate you through your approach towards taking anxiety's presence in your life. Stay tuned!

FIVE

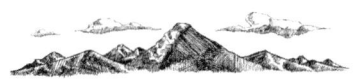

Acceptance and Approach

So, we're getting a grip on anxiety in this book. We're not making anxiety disappear. That's a pretty unrealistic expectation because of the fact that anxiety is a universal human emotion. In this chapter, we will work on accepting the struggle of life and its anxiety. We will look at skills we can develop to overcome anxiety, our self-talk when it comes to anxiety, and how we can adjust our approach and mindset towards anxiety to limit the damaging effects of unruly anxiety.

The Skill to Overcome Anxiety

Most therapists will tell you that eliminating anxiety symptoms isn't the same as removing the etiology. Just a fancy word for the cause or reason behind something of it. So I need to just take a minute to underline that in this book, we will be mostly focusing on limiting and managing the symptoms of general anxiety. Underlying serious psychological causes for anxiety, like trauma, might not heal through the strategies and management techniques shared in this book. Deep-rooted anxiety on the clinical spectrum requires longer-term psychotherapy under the guidance of a professional. But don't underestimate the value of developing skills and techniques to manage your general anxieties.

As we journey through this book, you'll all the more come to realize that you will probably never really overcome anxiety. However, you can overcome the obstacle of anxiety, ruining your life when you take the driver's seat, and manage how you engage with anxiety. Anxiety is a common human emotion that all people experience to some degree. To create the belief that you will completely overcome any form of anxiety in your life is not feasible. You can, however, overcome its potential to spiral out of control. Now that that's out of the way let's get into skills and techniques you can work on to manage the effects of anxiety in your everyday life.

Learn to manage your body and be aware of the mind-body relationship.

Make sure you fuel your body with nutrient-dense foods. Keep your body moving by introducing exercise into your everyday routine. It doesn't even need to be intense exercise. A simple 30-minute walk in nature or a few yoga stretches can do wonders (we'll get a little deeper into that later in the book).

Practice mindful awareness.

Realize that you don't always have to listen to the little voice of worry that calls. As you know by now, your amygdala stores some memories of past threatening experiences, and it might lead to some "false alarms." Take notice of how the "voice" manifests in your body. You'll often experience the voice in the form of dread. Usually, this is just a manifestation of physical tension. Acknowledge that the pressure is in your stomach, for example, and then use this feeling of tension for cueing a relaxation state for yourself. A few deep breaths can do wonders here. But I won't be sharing too many details on breath-work here because we've got a whole section dedicated to that later on. Take note that if you hear the voice of worry calling. Instead of allowing yourself to get enveloped in worry, use the voice as an indication of where you are manifesting tension. Call on a method to relax the parts of your being that need soothing. If you do this, you realize that worrying is a habit with a neurobiological connection to anxiety. If you believe worry is a sign of doom, you will find a cause for doom or dread and completely miss the opportunity to disarm some piled up tension.

Allow yourself to feel your anger.
I find this skill is one that is rarely discussed when anxiety is tabled. Suppressed anger can be a significant cause of anxiety. We tend to have a very negative connection to anger. So we suppress it and often don't even realize that it is actually anger we are feeling. This leads to frustration, but we can't pinpoint what we are so frustrated about. When you are feeling frustrated and angry, it might be a good idea to ask yourself if something happened that you might feel outraged about. Perhaps you didn't get that promotion, or maybe you have a partner with unhealthy spending habits. We're conditioned not to show anger to people or situations around us. But it doesn't mean that we don't feel anger on the inside.

By asking yourself whether you are angry and if you are angry, what you might be angry about, you indirectly open yourself to experience the anger without a negative outward display. Try writing the issues you are angry about on a piece of paper and physically throwing it away or even have a burning ritual if you feel like it. By acknowledging and releasing your anger, you can prevent it from manifesting as anxiety.

Learn to let your hair down and have some fun.
An old Japanese proverb says, "Time spent laughing is time spent with the Gods." When we genuinely laugh, we are almost transported to a different realm.

Laughter increases good feelings, and it's a great way to release tension. When people struggle with anxiety, they tend to take life very seriously and often need to relearn the ability to intentionally create fun. Work and play are equally important values to practice. When we stop experiencing humorous moments, we position ourselves to perceive everything as a potential problem. We restrain how we feel joy and delight. With the pace we are living these days, we tend to get so focused on slaying our goals that we forget what we like to do for fun. When anxiety lurks, take a moment to ask yourself when you last did something fun for yourself. Do you even know what you like to do for fun, and what makes you laugh?

Kick the habit of rumination and teach yourself to switch off and clear space.

Some people just have naturally ruminative brains. They're great at being rational and looking at many different angles. This can be a blessing, but also a great curse when anxiety creeps in. Sometimes, your own sanity must flip the switch and clear some space in your mind. An excellent visualization exercise to try here is to close your eyes and focus your thoughts on an open container image, ready to receive any of the many thoughts in your head. Name all of the thoughts hovering around the empty container. Visualize yourself, putting these thoughts into the box, and put a lid on it. Place the jar out of the way. Once the jar is out of the way, ask your mind if there is anything else left in your headspace outside of the jar. What is the most important current feeling or thought that surfaces in the space you are in? If you're at work, go to the jar and take out the one thing you named that relates to work. Give that your only focus. The rest of the jar can wait on the shelf until you move into a space where you can focus on the relevant issue. It's also a good idea to take out one peaceful thought to focus on before you go to bed. The goal here is to silence the overflow of thinking so that the reflective mind can rest and calm down.

Another technique that is great at managing the disruptive nature of rumination is the "Let's do it" method, which we get into later. But basically, when you are overwhelmed with thoughts, it disrupts the flood of thought by grabbing one issue from the thought-jar and applying the Let' s-Do-It technique. Take one small action towards the lingering issue in your mind.

Learn to plan so you can curb your worries.

If you tend to get distracted by thoughts and worries that cause you to struggle in prioritizing what really needs attention, you need to get a game plan in place for yourself. Some people have an innate knack for being decisive. Still, people who tend to ruminate can get really anxious about not prioritizing what needs to be done. The tricky thing is that over thinkers will overthink a plan. Even the most fail-proof idea in their mind can be hacked by the thought of another, seemingly better solution. So here's what you've got to do if your overthinking is continuously leading to anxiety:

- Step 1: Sit down and clearly and concretely define your problem.
- Step 2: Write a list of the options you have to solve the problem you are addressing.
- Step 3: Pick only one of the solutions on your options list.
- Step 4: Write an action plan for the chosen solution only and stick to it.

If your solution isn't working, adapt it. But do not go back to the other solutions. If you need to put those other solutions in your mind, jar, do it. If you don't stick to this, you run the risk of repeating a cycle of endless replanning. Sometimes getting something done is better than perfectly planning how you will reach the perfect solution. Ironically you get stuck in a space where you become great at planning but suck at execution. And let's be honest, a plan is only as good as it is executed. So just do it!

SIX

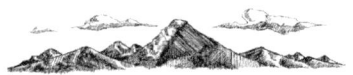

What to Tell Yourself to Overcome Anxiety and Panic Attacks

OFTEN ONE OF THE BIGGEST INSTIGATORS OF ANXIETY IS THE conversation we have with ourselves. Even a lack of communication with yourself can be a great igniter of anxiety because then we remain in a reactive state and not a conscious state.

But where and how do I start these conversations to engage my higher brain through consciousness?

Below are some general statements that illustrate how the reactive, instinctive brain may communicate, versus a conscious way of communicating through the higher brain. If you can get to a point where you are aware of the kind of messaging that can trigger anxiety or set off a panic attack, you can use these conscious comebacks by choice. Empower your higher brain to feel content.

My Anxiety Speaking Through My Limbic System and Lower Brain
My Higher Brain Speaking with Consciousness

A. I can't do this. I'll never get this task finished in time.

I might struggle with this task, but as I struggle, I will be learning and know how to complete similar tasks better in the future. Each intimidating thing I complete becomes less intimidating the next time I attempt it.

B. I keep failing at things and having to start over from nothing.
I learn from my failures, and I now start my journey from experience and not from scratch.

C. Everyone keeps asking things from me and I can't say no and I can't keep up with the pressure.
I am allowed to say "no".
No. (This is a complete sentence!). I do not have to explain my boundaries to anyone. I control how much pressure I'm going to allow into my life.

D. People are out to criticize everything I do and there is no room for mistakes in this world.
Not everything I do means something to the people around me and mistakes are a part of my learning process.

E. The world is filled with panic and chaos.
I have limitless access to calm, peace, and clarity.

F. I feel like I always have to explain myself and my actions.
I realize that I am growing into a higher consciousness when I don't have to explain myself because I am learning about myself daily.

. . .

G. My schedule is overbooked to the point where I'm constantly exhausted.

I scheduled time for myself to rest and meditate on positive thoughts when needed because I cannot be of value in this world if I do not practice self-care.

H. I'm tired of spending energy on people who do not meet any of my needs and it makes me feel unworthy of being loved.

I accept that people are limited by their own unresolved trauma. I practice self-loving and forgive myself for the times I belittle myself.

I. This situation is overwhelming so I lash out or dissociate.

I am practicing self-observation in overwhelming situations and learn what triggers anxiety in my being.

J. I can't get anything right. I'm a stupid nobody.

It's ok to feel overwhelmed. Sometimes life throws you a curveball. Breathe. I am human. I am alive. I am enough.

K. I feel so embarrassed. I should just crawl into a hole and never show my face again.

It's ok, I was nervous. I was brave enough to try something. Next time I will do better.

Counterintuitive Questions You Can Practice When You're Anxious

Let's face it. When you're in the midst of a panic attack or enveloped with anxiety, some of the most harmful things you can hear from someone is, "just let it go." Or maybe "stop being so negative," "just practice a little gratitude," or "just stop worrying." It should be pretty clear that anxiety can be completely irrational and really hard to calm.

These days we have so much access to information on anxiety. It almost seems that people believe it to be as simple as taming and calming some wild animals. We hear, see, and read that anxiety can be unhealthy. This leads to a fear of this emotion when, actually, it is just another emotion and should be treated as such. Let's take a step backward and simplify the relationship we have with this emotion: let's face it head-on. Just as we would face love, joy, hate, or any other emotion. Instead of dissecting anxiety further, let's look at a counterintuitive approach, where we embrace our anxiety instead of fighting it.

When anxiety surfaces, try interrupting your instinctive FFF-responses with these questions:

Hello Anxiety, is that you? What are you trying to show me today?

Often when we feel anxious, we rush into an impulsive, mindless, and soothing mood. When you feel a sporadic urge to do something out of the blue, like watching a series immediately or grabbing something unhealthy from the fridge to gobble down. Stop to ask where this is coming from. Ask if it is anxiety in disguise. Have a chat with yourself to determine whether you are starving, or if you are actually trying to fulfill a need inside of you that you are anxious about. When we feel anxious, it is often accompanied by a level of discomfort. Let's be honest: we humans do not like to be in uncomfortable situations. But this discomfort is actually your body asking you to pay attention to something, through anxiety. So welcome the anxiety and ask it why it has shown up instead of numbing it away with a mindless form of soothing.

Dear Senses, what are you five whispering about Anxiety at this moment?

By asking your senses about the way they are experiencing anxiety, you call on the mind and body approach by taking stock of your relationship to a specific environment. In doing this, you are not fighting anxiety, but getting to know it intimately.

What am I hearing that makes me anxious? Is the sound of traffic outside making me anxious? Would it be a good idea to invest in a quality headset to silence out some noise?

What am I seeing that makes me anxious? Start naming things one by one that makes you anxious. This aids in calming you down and getting you present in your body.

Am I tasting something odd in my mouth due to a chemical reaction, or did a specific taste trigger some feeling of anxiety? Perhaps the taste of chicken soup irritates you, so you just eat more and more of it. But actually, the taste reminded you of the loss of your mother. The chicken soup triggered a fond memory of her.

What am I feeling? Is the touch of something physically irritating me? Perhaps I'm tactilely sensitive and need to pay more attention to the textiles of the clothes I'm purchasing. Do I feel uncomfortable about the way someone touches me? Perhaps I should communicate some healthy boundaries regarding the way I'm allowing this person to touch me.

What am I smelling? Is it the smell of the cologne of a person passing by that reminded me of an ex? Maybe I still have some unresolved feelings of loss I need to attend to.

At the very least, these inviting, counterintuitive questions will break up a painful or negative thought pattern. It will make you realize that you are not anxious, but you have anxiety in you. Your anxiety isn't defining you, it could just be guiding you into some new insights.

Choosing What Thoughts to Weigh in On

It is not only our internal conversations we need to pay attention to when approaching our anxiety. We also need to choose the thoughts we spend our energy on.

One of the most well-known symptoms of anxiety is that of racing thoughts. Often, these thoughts are both fleeting and repetitive in pattern. They can surface as a single issue or as multiple different lines of thought. For example, you may have racing thoughts about your partner, who is suddenly working late every night. This is one issue you focus on, but this can escalate into multiple chains of thinking: "Am I being insecure?", "Is he or she being unfaithful?" "If my partner is unfaithful, how will I handle that?", "Will the betrayal break me?" and "What if they're not being unfaithful? Will I then be considered an ungrateful jealous partner?" Oh, and the list can go on and on.

When you have racing thoughts, you may experience:

- Difficulty in focusing on anything else.
- An inability to "switch off" and relax.
- A feeling of helplessness because you can't slow down your thoughts.
- How you catastrophize all kinds of worst-case scenarios.
- Insomnia.

So what do I do to manage my thoughts when they spiral?

Create a mantra for yourself. It can be something as straightforward as, "This too shall pass." It just gives you a way to stop the spiral and focus your mind on the mantra. Keep repeating the mantra while taking relaxed breaths and focus on your mantra until your mind, too, comes to a halt.

Ensure you get a relaxing routine in place before you go to

bed. Racing thoughts just love getting into bed with you - but in no sexy manner will it keep you awake. If you do not deliberately attempt to relax your body and mind at least one to two hours before bed, you're bound to have your subconscious mind wake you at all unusual hours of the night. You will wake up sleepy, stressed, and with no energy. Drink some chamomile tea, switch off the television, and all screens to reduce your blue light exposure. A few yoga stretches can go a long way. Read a relaxing book, not one that gets your thoughts too engaged. Take a great Epsom salt bath and add some lavender or any one of your favorite essential oils. And do yourself a big favor and invest in a $10.00 old school bedside alarm. Put your phone on charge in the hallway, kitchen, or anywhere out of sight. If you are anxious about missing an emergency call, adjust your phone's settings to allow specific contacts' notifications to come through. This brings me to my next point, and golly, it was a game-changer for me.

Get off the phone, George! Gee whiz. Smartphones have changed our lives for the positive. But they are flawed in many ways in terms of the way we interact with them. When advising on getting the smartphone out of the bedroom, it wasn't just to prevent the notifications from waking you and avoiding the impulse to browse social media, etc. Have you ever thought about it? Your smartphone is the last thing you embrace before you go to bed, and the first thing you touch when you wake up. Come on. And when you wake, what do you do if you don't hit the snooze button? You start checking every little notification on your phone. So what about it? Well, basically, your emails and social media are means of communication. When you unlock that screen and start scrolling, you're basically letting all those into your bed before you've even had coffee or a cup of tea! Would you respond to your boss if he/she called you while still in bed? No. So why are you doing it via email?

You're in bed with your boss! It might sound a tad exaggerated - but is it really?

Science shows that our cortisol (the stress hormone) levels are highest in the morning. Instead of doing something to reduce it, you raise the level by letting other people's thoughts and requests into your bed before you've said good morning to your kids or your dog for that matter. Do yourself a favor, and for one week, try it. Just put the phone outside and take at least one hour before you expose yourself to everything on that smart little box. Embrace your partner after killing the old school alarm. Get up and do 15-20 reps of a light exercise - just until you break a little sweat. Once the sweat breaks, you've basically halved your cortisol levels. Take a few minutes tho breathe and meditate on your mantra. And then go wake the kids or feed the dog or connect with something that feeds your soul. See, now you can at least feel you did something for yourself before all the world's requests infiltrate your day. If you let the world in on your phone too early, you're already allowing other thoughts to weigh in on your life before considering how you are feeling.

Essentially, when our anxious thoughts are racing, the gist of the exercise is to create space for calm and simplicity. If you cannot manage that, you will most likely only feel anxiety, fear, or overwhelmedness. Any underlying emotions or thoughts will be overridden by these big three emotions.

It really is by no means as simple as "letting go of worries and negative emotions." One needs to create a safe space to process your thoughts before deciding which thoughts are relevant and deserve attention.

SEVEN

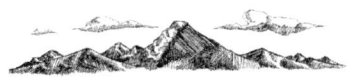

Pushing Anxiety Over the Edge

We can push anxiety over the edge by getting strategies before she surfaces with her dark side.

A Strategy for Mindfulness

When you feel your thoughts spiraling out of control, take a few minutes to pull yourself towards yourself and your current surroundings. Practice mindfulness by turning your focus to the present. Come back into your body. Find something in the environment that grounds you in the present moment. When you are present, your thoughts are steered away from the past, and the future and anxiety starts to subside.

When you are present in the moment, you can feel the aliveness in your body now. And realize that all you have is now. The past is a place we should learn from, not a place to call home.

Get your triggers into a lineup!

Make a list of situations and people that make you feel anxious. Get them out on a piece of paper, so it's like a lineup. Then have a good look at each culprit. See what they look like and how they disguise themselves so that when you go out into the world, you know what these culprits look like, and you can never be caught or harassed by them. And if they do show up, know that you are armed with the necessary weapons to fight them off and create a safe zone for yourself. For example, if you are anxious to talk to people over the phone, don't let the list of calls your boss just handed out to make you anxious. See it as an opportunity to arm yourself with the ability to build up resilience against the anxiety braided into the task at hand. The discomfort will fade with time, and soon you'll be able to pop into your boss's office and ask if you can make any calls on his behalf! We can only banish the devils we know.

The Let's Do It Technique

"Birds do it.
Bees do it.
Even educated fleas do it.
Let's do it... let's... consciously disrupt our anxious thoughts!"

Remember, in Chapter 1, we spoke about the three brain regions. How do we, as humans, have the unique ability to consciously experience things through our higher brain because of our choices?

Well, that's why we developed the "Let's Do It Technique."

Every time you find yourself faced with some sort of feeling of anxiety, I want you to engage with the consciousness in your higher brain. Disrupt the overwhelming thoughts sprouting from your limbic system and lower brain's physical reactions, by saying: "Let's Do It!"

But what exactly are we doing? You are engaging a team effort between your three brain regions, intending to reset the instinctive fight, flee, or freeze reaction to perceived threats. We are disrupting negative feelings and thoughts like:

- "I'll never be able to do push-ups."

- "I can't have a difficult conversation with my spouse."
- "I will never get out of debt."

And through our higher brain, we use the phrase "Let's Do It" to navigate these thoughts into small empowering acts that build up resilience to the paralyzing or avoiding effects of anxiety. We change our narrative to:

"Let's do it. Just one wall push-up. Then a few more. Let's just do it. I might not be able to do push-ups yet. But let's do it".

"Let's do it. I'll share a smaller difficult issue with my spouse and take it from there. I am deeply loved by my spouse. So all three regions of the brain, let's do it!'

"Let's do it. Let's get out of debt. Let's get a second job. Let's set up a budget. Let's do it."

One of the significant problems with anxiety is that we get so wrapped up in our minds that we do not even think about doing anything. When you just commit to doing something seemingly insignificant for at least five minutes, chances are you'll continue working on it. When we are overwhelmed by anxiety, we get so caught up in potential scenarios that tend to escalate to much more significant proportions in our minds. We become unable to see any starting point to tackle an issue at hand. It's like the old African proverb asking how you eat an elephant? One bite at a time.

By disrupting our spiraling thoughts of "oh this is too great to handle," or "I can't even comprehend a solution," you pull your feelings towards the present by saying, "let's do it." This can be the first, small practical action you can take in the situation. You do not have to have the whole future repercussions of your little action planned out. No one on Earth has that kind of power or control. The future will always have some sort of uncertainty involved. The future also isn't always far away. It's literally a second away. As each second is ticking by, the future is happening. By changing your narrative to "let's do it," where it is the first thing you do in the present, you draw your attention away from past and future events.

Use Your Imagination

First of all, we need to be honest with each other. Some of us just let our vivid imaginations run wild when it comes to anxious situations. Can you relate? If I were to give you a moment to fool around with an idea, you'd probably spin off into a roller coaster ride of anxiety. This crazy adrenaline rushing trip takes you absolutely nowhere!

But wait, if you have a vivid imagination, don't get too dreary now. Remember, we have the gift of neuroplasticity - the ability to rewind our minds into a calm space. We can do this through guided visualization and imagery. However, before we get into that, I'd like to share the story of Susanna with you.

Susanna Forest is the author of The Age of the Horse: An Equine Journey through History. She shared a powerful example of the role imagination can play in anxiety and fear during an interview with Bridget Kendall on BBC (2016) through her own personal experience.

Susanna refers to how she used her imagination in horse riding as a child, versus how she applied her imagination as an adult.

She describes that as a child, she was fearless in respect to horses. She mainly focused her imagination on nice things like imagining having a hundred Arab horses and winning the grand national horse race. However, as an adult, she started using the same imagination to think about terrible things that didn't necessarily come to pass.

So as an adult, she created an artificial construction that

wasn't really based on anything in the real environment of fear. It was built psychologically through her imagination.

Isn't this just a great example of how powerful our imaginations can be? However, our power lies in the way we apply our imagination.

The question is, are we applying our imaginations as Forest did as a little girl? Imagining nice things (and by the way, those nice things she imagined, manifested in her life's work with and through horses)? Or, are we applying our imagination like the adult version of Forest? Through a focus on all the bad things that could happen?

Guided Visualization and Imagery

We can use our imaginations to guide ourselves into a place of relaxation and peace. With this technique, we train our minds to go to a pleasant, serene milieu filled with beauty. When you use your imagination here, it's essential to utilize all five senses. As you imagine a space, you need to see, hear, smell, and even taste it!

For example, the space that I guide myself to is my little patch of grass in my backyard. This is the place where I will sit barefoot and fell the grass between my toes. The Sun is filtered by the palm trees which have grown so much since I first planted them. The scent is always slightly haunted by the smell of the damp soil in the humidity in Florida. I hear the Florida Scrub Jay (yes, an actual bird) calling in the grapefruit tree. The gentle morning sun drips warmth upon my face. This is where I feel most at peace. I sit up straight on the steps with my hands upon my knees. When I feel overwhelmed by a situation, I position myself in the same position, I would sit upon those steps. I close my eyes. By visualizing the space in my imagination, my body is also led to believe we are in that calm space because my position reminds it of residing in that realm of calm.

When a breathing exercise isn't enough to soothe your

anxiety into a relaxed state, try a little combo with your imagination.

To get started, work through the instructions and answer the questions below.

Self-Awareness Exercise

How to use my imagination and senses to guide myself into a realm of calm.

1. Locate a comfortable place where you can sit or lie down.
2. Loosen any tight shoes or clothing items that might be causing strain or tension in your body.
3. Shut your eyes and take in a few deep breaths.
4. Think of a place in nature where you encountered deep calm and serenity. Maybe it's the beach? A lake? The mountains? The desert?
5. What do you see with your mind's eye?
6. What do you smell with your mind's eye?
7. What do you taste with your mind's eye?
8. What do you feel with your mind's eye?
9. What do you hear with your mind's eye?

Visual imagery can enhance a state of anxiety when applied to anticipated disasters and doom that invade our thoughts. It is essential to notice that we are relaxed whenever we are in a relaxed state. Then bring your attention to your surroundings. The goal is to sharpen your senses and discover the details in your surroundings that make you feel calm and relaxed. Notice the colors around you, the textures, shapes, positioning of your surroundings, and the proportion. Are the large trees majestic or intimidating? Is the texture of the chair cover soothing or scratching? Is the sound of the water empowering or agitating?

You can see that these experiences are deeply personal. You need to take time to get to know your sensual preferences and details that are conducive to the management of your specific anxieties. While huge trees are calming to me, it might be overwhelming and a cause of nightmare for the person next to me. Waves might calm one person but make another feel as they might drown. By getting to know what exactly calms us in scenarios, we can easily guide our imaginations to harness our minds and bodies into the spaces where we feel calm and safe. If your images are vague, your calming response will be unclear.

A few things to keep in mind when attempting the utilization of your imagination:

- Keep things enjoyable - this should be fun!
- Let your creativity flow when creating your feel-good scenes. You can have more than one scene in your "imagination's archive." The cottage in the canyon is a big favorite. Still, when I need comfort more than relaxation, I envision the old coal stove on my grandparents' farm. I used to sit there, warming up a newborn lamb that lost its mother. The smell of the fire in the stove, the warmth is building up between myself and the soft wool of the little lamb. Oh, I can go into every little detail. But that moment not only calms, but it comforts! So build up your archive!
- Expand your descriptive vocabulary. Remember, in Chapter 2, I referred to the frustration people have due to a limited emotional vocabulary? Well, the same goes for the imagination exercise. If you build up a vocabulary to express your senses' details, you're in for a treat! When thinking up and working on your imaginary archive of calming spaces, consider having a thesaurus nearby.
- Make peace with the fact that there is no 'right' or

'wrong' in this exercise. You shouldn't judge the scenes you are creating.
- Try adding reassuring affirmations in your scenes like: "I'm feeling calmer and comforted." "I feel my worries blowing away in the breeze." or "My body is starting to release tension and getting looser and looser."

This is one of my own favorite means of getting a grip on my anxiety. However, if this is not your vibe, don't worry. There are other tools to assist you in gaining a firmer grip.

EIGHT

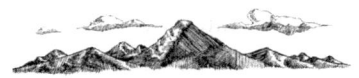

How to Feel Safe Wherever You Are

It's no mystery that people who grapple with anxiety tend to feel doomed, dreary, unsafe. As if someone or something is out to get them. But that's not really true. It's just how your brain has been conditioned in terms of safety. Here's some golden advice for rewiring your brain to make you feel safe wherever you go.

Zero- to Neuro: Utilizing Neuroplasticity to Train Your Mind to Feel Safe

In Pittman & Karle's book Rewire Your Anxious Brain (2015), they highlight "the promise of neuroplasticity." Now you are probably wondering what neuroplasticity is and how the hell it relates to feeling safe wherever you are, right?

In neuroscience, the term "neuroplasticity" refers to the brain's incredible ability to change its neuro-pathways and its patterns of reaction. Pittmann and Karle referenced Taub's work. Taub found that people whose brains were damaged by strokes could actually be taught to use different parts of their brains to move their arms again. Furthermore, under certain circumstances, the circuits in our brains responsible for sight can develop the capacity to respond to sound within a few days.

Furthermore, the brain can develop new connections in straightforward ways. For example, some research shows that merely thinking about taking specific actions, like playing a particular song on the guitar or hitting that hole in one on the golf course, can literally lead to changes in the region of the brain that controls those movements.

Basically, "the promise of neuroplasticity" means that the brain isn't stagnant or fixed. Nor is it unchangeable. This also implies that your brain's circuits or neuro-pathways aren't just genetically passed on. Still, they are formed through the things we experience, how we behave, and the way we think.

But what has this all got to do with feeling safe in any place you happen to be?

Look, instead of showing you a list of small items you can try, I want to provide you with this powerful piece of knowledge. If you feel anxious because your neuro-pathways have been shaped by experiences where you have been lead to believe that you are never safe and secure, you can rest in the promise of neuroplasticity. It is not ever too soon or too late for you to begin working on rewiring your brain's circuitry. To be resistant to fear and attracted to feelings of safety, security, and belonging.

If you believe yourself to be quite high on the spectrum of anxiety disorders, it might be a good idea to seek the guidance of a cognitive-behavioral therapist who specializes in more advanced techniques in the field. However, if you just have mild cases of anxious experiences, there is a lot of self-work you can do.

NINE

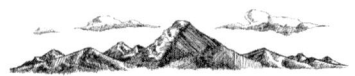

How to Deal With a Fear of Failure

BY NOW, WE KNOW THAT WHEN OUR AMYGDALA DETECTS A threat, we can experience a great sense of fear as an immediate response. This fear can have an intense paralyzing effect - sometimes to the extent that our fear of what might happen prevents us from taking action in any way. We just avoid whatever leads or relates to the trigger of fear. In this section, we look at failure as a trigger for fear.

Have you ever been confronted with such an intense fear of failing at something? That you just altogether avoid trying whatever it is you think you might fail at? Most people have probably experienced this at one time or another. If we allow our fear response to the failure to stop us from moving forward in our lives, we run a considerable risk of missing opportunities for more significant development along our life's journey.

What are potential triggers or causes for fear of failure?

Before we can determine what triggers our fear of failure, we need to find out what 'failure' means. People have various interpretations of what they consider failure. Why is this? Because we all have different backgrounds, benchmarks, belief systems, and end values shaped in us. What might be perceived as a significant failure to one person might be nothing more than a simple learning experience to another.

Practically every human is afraid of failing at some stage in their life. How often this might happen or how great the extent of fear of failure stretches is rooted in how we perceive our failings. Our perceptions are significantly formed due to past experiences. Especially while growing up. For instance, if, as a child, you had very critical parents who set unrealistic expectations of your capabilities, you might be a constant 'failure-fearer'. This is because you would have been undermined continuously in any attempt you made at reaching for the expectation your parents set out for you. These negative feelings of powerlessness, incompetence, and unworthiness will very likely follow you well into adulthood.

Exposure to a profoundly traumatic event at some intersection of life (not only in childhood) may also trigger you to be a 'failure-fearer.' For example, say you had to do a presentation at work in front of the whole office, and you didn't do very well. This feeling of shame, humiliation, and feeling downright dumb could be experienced as so destructive to your self-esteem that you developed a fear of failing at other things at work and in your personal life too. You might still be walking around with those feelings for years and years later.

How do I know if I am experiencing fear of failure?

If you are uncertain if you just have a little nervousness about attempting something, or are edging close to a "fear-failure-mindset", here are some symptoms of people who genuinely fear failure:

A *reluctance* to make an attempt at a new project or skill.

- You indulge in *self-sabotage* through procrastination, showing no follow through on

your goals, allowing yourself to feel always anxious and avoiding anything that might feel slightly uncomfortable.
- You lean into **perfectionism** to the extent that you will only attempt things that you know you can complete successfully, quickly, and perfectly.
- **Self-confidence** is something utterly foreign to you. you find yourself using negative phrases like "I'll never be a part of that team because I'm not smart enough," "I'll never be pretty enough to be loved," and "I'll never be good enough to get promoted at work."

If you find yourself engaging with any of the mentioned behaviors, you might want to invest in a little perception-based strategy to manage your fear of failure.

Defining what failure means to me.

As I said, the glorious thing about failure is that we can define what it means to us. We can choose how we perceive failure: as the end of the world and proof that we are incredibly inadequate or as a marvelous learning experience. When we fail at something, a tremendous immediate response is to ask yourself: what can I learn from this? Failures are embedded with valuable lessons that help us grow and prevent us from making the same mistakes. Failure can only stop you if you allow it to.

Check it out. So many people experienced failure but rose above it, learned from it and triumphed:

- **Michael Jordan** was cut from his high school basketball team. He missed more than 9,000 shots, and on 26 occasions, he was trusted to make the winning shot, and he missed. Yet he is still one of the greatest basketball players of all time. Jordan has repeatedly said that he has failed over and over

in his life. That his failures are the reasons for his success.
- **Steven Spielberg** was rejected two times by the University of Southern California's School of Cinematic Arts. He kept at it, and by 2019, his cinematic output grossed over $9 billion. He also won three Academy Awards.
- The author, **JK Rowling**, known for the Harry Potter novels, was on welfare, divorced, depressed, a single mother, and wrote her first novel while studying. She was rejected by twelve publishers before she reached success and is now one of the world's richest women.
- **Jerry Seinfeld** was a young comedian before his famous TV-show. His first time on stage sucked. His freeze-reaction kicked in, and the crowd started to 'boo' him off the stage. Seinfeld could have let his fear of failing a second time get the better of him and just pack up and convince himself that comedy wasn't in the cards. Instead, he got on the same stage the following night, and the audience cried from laughter. Today he is deemed one of the most successful comedians of all time.
- **Elvis Presley** was told that he would go nowhere and that he ought to be driving a truck after his first performance at the Grand Ole Opry. Despite this seemingly failed performance, Presley did not fear failure to get the best of him. He turned into one of the world's greatest stars with a legacy that shines to this day.

This list can continue forever, but are you getting the swing of things? You need to sit with yourself. Make a serious call as to how you will define your failures. Or are you going to let failure define you?

Most often, our most valuable insights follow our greatest failures. How will you ever discover how strong and capable you are if you never fall, get up, and try again? How will you know who your real friends are who will motivate you when you are struggling if you never allow yourself some struggle?

Practical ways to minimize your fear of failing.

Once you've cleared up how you define and perceive failure, you will feel empowered to face the chance of failing and see it as a courageous act that will lead to a fuller life. This perception change won't happen overnight, though. It will take some practice and commitment. So here are some practical tips for you to reduce your fear of failure.

Map potential outcomes.

A large number of people fear the unknown. By drawing up a map of potential outcomes of an action or decision, you will minimize the fear of the unknown and feel more secure.

Practice positive thinking and self-conversation.

Through practicing kind self-talk and positive thinking, you build your self-confidence and quiet your own inner-critic. This action also aids in neutralizing self-sabotage.

Welcome the worst-case-scenario.

When we welcome the worst-case-scenario, we might actually realize that it isn't so bad after all. On the flip side, it may be genuinely catastrophic. Still, you will have peace in that your fear is perfectly rational and sharpens your ability to recognize rational vs. irrational fear of failure.

Have "Plan B" in place.

If you have a backup plan in place, or a second direction to try out, you might feel less of a 'sting' from your failure because you know you have another option to explore. This failure isn't the proverbial end for you.

Don't just set goals, set small and SMART goals.

If someone has a fear of failure, big goals and dreams

might just seem too darn far away and out of reach. So when you set goals for yourself, or when someone is setting them on your behalf, say at work, use small and SMART principles to compartmentalize your goals. This strategy will help you gain "small wins." It will lead to a sense of accomplishment that releases dopamine. Dopamine is a neurotransmitter that works with brain chemicals, much like serotonin, oxytocin, and endorphins. It plays a vital role in how happy our bodies feel.

A small goal is a small goal. If you feel like you will never be able to lose weight, don't start by cutting sugar, cutting refined carbs, and working out five times a week. Take one small step towards the goal. Start by just cutting out sugar. Once you've got that under wraps. Celebrate the small victory and go on to the next goal: cutting out refined carbs. Then go from there. You with me?

But what is a SMART goal? Does it wear fancy shoes? No silly, it's an abbreviation for Specific, Measurable, Attainable, Relevant, and Time-bound.

When you set your eyes on a goal, it's not only a good idea to break it down into smaller goals, but you also need to ask if the goal is realistically set out. If I want to lose 50 pounds in a month, my goal isn't set up realistically. Let me show you what a smart goal can look like vs. an unrealistic goal where you are setting yourself up for failure.

A goal setting you up for failure:

I am going to lose 50 pounds in one month.

Specific? Not really.

Measurable? Yes.

Attainable? No.

Relevant? No, if set in this way, expected results will not be reliable or reasonable.

Time-bound? Though time is connected to the goal, it is not realistic.

A goal set up in the SMART way:

I am going to lose 50 pounds in 22 weeks. My intention is

to lose 2-3 pounds per week. I will do this by seeking support from a dietician to set up a meal plan for weight loss individuals to my body's needs. I will steadily introduce moderate, pleasant exercise into my weekly routine. I will exercise a minimum of 3 days per week for at least 30 minutes.

Specific? Yes.
Measurable? Yes.
Attainable? Yes.
Relevant? Yes.
Time-bound? Yes.

See the difference here? Which of these two goals would you most likely reach? Which of these goals eases your fear of failure?

Fundamentally, this whole section on how to deal with a fear of failure aims to help you realize you are not the only person fearing failure. Every human being will experience this fear at some stage of our lives, but we should not allow our fear to hinder us from progressing.

Regardless of the cause of your fear, you must never forget that you have a higher brain that enables you to choose how you will react to whatever triggers your fear of failure. You can choose to see it as an obstacle that is too big to overcome, or an opportunity to step-up and grow into a stronger, more confident version of yourself.

How to No Longer Care What People Think of You

The main goal of this book is to get a grip on anxiety so that you are empowered to live your life authentically.

However, we cannot truly live and love authentically if we keep comparing ourselves to others. There's a quote by Lao Tzu that says if you care about what other people think, you will always be their prisoner. I really couldn't have said it better myself. Maybe I could have, but this links so perfectly with one of the key things we struggle with when it comes to anxiety. We already imprison ourselves in our own heads, now like that's not enough, we go and allow ourselves to be further imprisoned in the heads of other people.

The simple truth is: other people's thoughts and opinions have everything to do with them, and absolutely nothing to do with us. You have no idea what their neuro-pathways look like from their past experiences. You have no idea what they could be projecting onto you. And remember this darling, anxiety is probably the most contagious emotion of all. If you're already prone to anxiety, take extra care when you detect other people's anxieties spiraling out of control because you might catch it. Again.

But is it just as simple as "not caring"? How do you get to such a point when the need to feel accepted? To feel like we belong is so hardwired into our systems?

There's no harm done when you feel like you want to belong. Still, when your need to be accepted by others becomes more significant than your self-acceptance, things become a problem. When we start analyzing every single glance in our direction and interpret it as a form of judgment when someone passes by you without greeting you, you may become convinced that you are not worth being noticed. When we are continually trying to please everyone around us… we don't only become exhausted. We are not practicing a healthy balance between acceptance by others and our self-acceptance and self-worth.

So what can you practically do to get yourself in a position of authenticity and no longer giving a hoot about what others think of you?

If you recognize yourself as a person who tends to be anxious about being liked and genuinely concerned with others' opinions, here are some tips to help you step into a healthier relationship with yourself and others:

Know your worth and your values.
If you don't know your value, you'll settle for anything the

world offers. It's like having a vintage watch that might be worth a great deal. Still, if you don't know its worth or fight for its fair value, you'll probably sell it to a pawn shop instead of an avid antique collector.

Set, know, and practice your own boundaries.

If you don't tell people how to treat you and what you will or will not allow in your life, they'll handle you the way they like. Communicating boundaries may sound like: "I love having you here. I just don't appreciate it when you show up unannounced," "I don't mind lending you things. Still, please ask if you can borrow them before just taking them," "I understand that you are angry, but if you keep on yelling out of control I am walking out and taking space." Get it?

Keep things in perspective.

We tend to think people think of us all the time. But in reality, we all have more than enough to keep ourselves occupied with. If you meet someone new and you're worried about what they think of you, don't. They are probably doing exactly the same. That… or they're just running down the rest of their "to-do list" in the back of their minds.

Acknowledge that you have ownership of your own feelings

You do not have to base your feelings on other people's opinions or approval. You are allowed to feel that a Tom Waits song is beautiful when someone else tells you he hurts their ears with his off-pitch growling. We like different things. That's ok.

Question your own thinking.

Our brains are absolutely fascinating, oh, but they can be very deceitful at times. See, we humans tend to lean towards cognitive distortions and patterns that promote negative thinking. Think how often we assume the worst, or how quickly we jump to conclusions, or how (contradictory to what we do on Instagram) we filter out the beauty in a situation and only focus on what's nasty. Pay attention to your impulsive thoughts and question them to make sure you're not falling into a pattern of making the worst assumptions about a situation that only exists in your mind.

1. Ease up on perfectionism.
2. Know that your best is enough.
3. Remember that everyone makes mistakes.
4. We are all flawed, and we are all here to learn through our mistakes—no self-bullying required here.
5. Really get to know yourself.

Acknowledge that every human has a deep desire to belong. Some are just more prone to develop anxiety around acceptance and belonging. But before you shame yourself for not being good enough to join a book club, make sure you even enjoy reading. Or that you enjoy the kind of books the club reads. Or that you find the pace at which they read enjoyable. Maybe that book club isn't for you. Perhaps you actually prefer taking part in a book forum rather than drinking wine and gossiping, pretending that you read books. See, sometimes we get lost in not feeling good enough, where the debate was never around your worth, but rather, is this even what I like? Know yourself. And well, sometimes you have to also do something and not like it. Knowing what you don't like is a step closer to what you do like.

Once you find your vibe, find your tribe.

Once you get to know yourself and what you like, look for people who have the same vibe. Don't waste your time conforming to other people who don't radiate the same energy or interests as you. Circle yourself with people who actually appreciate you in all your wonderful authenticity.

Just accept a helping hand already.

If all of these techniques seem to fail you and you still seem overwhelmed by what others think of you, be kind to yourself. Accept that you might be sitting with some deep unresolved trauma or a mental health issue and seek the help and care you need. You do not have to try and be tough. You will just prolong your suffering, sweet human. Just don't.

You will never be able to make everyone like you, nor will you ever be like them ultimately. You can, however, get to know your value and worth in this world and hold on to that. You are enough, and you are so welcome in this world.

TEN

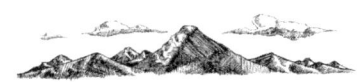

A Special on Panic Attacks
―――――――――――――――

Extra, extra! Read all about it! That's right, a special on panic attacks coming your way!

So we've mentioned panic attacks quite a few times throughout the book as symptoms of anxiety. But what is a panic attack? What is going on in our bodies when we have one? And what can we do to soften the blow when they surface?

Before we get into our special on panic attacks, let's just have a brief conversation about the distinction between an anxiety attack and a panic attack. In essence, they are the same thing, just under different conditions.

Anxiety attacks are not acknowledged in the Diagnostic and Statistical Manual of Mental Disorders. Anxiety itself is recognized as a part of several psychiatric disorders. An anxiety attack is slower in onset than a panic attack with less severe symptoms. In a nutshell, you can have an anxiety and panic attack at the same time.

Panic attacks are, however, recognized in the Diagnostic and Statistical Manual of Mental Disorders and are grouped into two categories: expected or unexpected.

Expected panic attacks occur as a reaction to a specific

trigger or stressor, like phobias. Unexpected panic attacks occur without an apparent cause. This is where the "attack" in "panic attack" becomes of the essence. An unexpected panic attack is a sudden, unpredictable, uncomfortable, frightening, and even painful occurrence. A panic attack is the body's most extreme anxiety reaction/manifestation.

Once a person starts to have regular panic attacks, they often feel helpless. They might not want to be left alone or be around public places. If left unmanaged, panic attack victims may keep on functioning in a state of physical and psychological tension, in anticipation and preparation for the next attack. Some therapists refer to this as anticipatory anxiety.

To better understand the make-up of a panic attack, we can refer back to the amygdala's fight, flee, or freeze response (FFF-response) to find a trigger. First, let's familiarize ourselves with some symptoms of panic attacks: trembling, dizziness, increased heart rate, shortness of breath or difficulty breathing normally, confusion, stomach distress, and an inability to focus. These symptoms are all connected to the amygdala's FFF-response. They can manifest in such a way that people think they are going nuts or having a stroke or heart attack. Symptoms of a panic attack generally culminate within the initial 10-20 minutes, but some might last hours. But if you understand that the root of your attack lies in your amygdala's response, doesn't it seem just a tad less intimidating?

Understand how your body reacts in emergency situations.

You also need to get this. When you are amid an FFF-response, it is entirely normal to feel like you're seeing yourself in an emergency situation rather than being able to consciously control how you respond. Why? Because your amygdala responds faster than your conscious brain, and it has the insane ability to override other brain processes. Mighty little almond we have got nestled in our brains.

When we discussed how our three brain regions function separately, yet we experience these functions as one? Cool. This comes into play when we take a more in-depth look at panic attacks too. Your amygdala has a lot of tiny connections to the higher brain (cortex). These many tiny connections allow the amygdala a significant amount of influence on the higher brain's response. The higher brain also has little connections running to the amygdala, but not nearly as many connections as the amygdala has running to the cortex. So you could literally say that your amygdala has a firmer 'grip' on the cortex than vice versa. It also means that when your amygdala takes the wheel, the poor old cortex needs to jump in the back. Basically, your thinking process within the cortex is temporarily suspended when the amygdala's got a spell on it.

When I realized this, for a moment, I questioned this "arrangement." How is that practical at all? You might ponder the same thing, so here goes: say you're in a public place. Someone pulls out a gun and just starts shooting, would it be wiser for your cortex to stand and analyze the caliber of the weapon, the expression on the gunman's face, or just to run for shelter? Do you now understand why some people can't remember details from a life-threatening situation?

When it comes to panic attacks (which are amygdala-based anxiety), it's essential to understand the amygdala's superpower of taking over. The brain is hardwired to provide the amygdala to briefly take over control in unsafe conditions. Because of this particular wiring set-up, it really is hard to use reason-based thought processes in your higher brain when a genuinely perceived threat is detected by the amygdala. For the same reason, people in a shooting can't always remember the shooter's face. Anxious people who suffer from a panic attack can often not recall some details in the offset of the attack.

The amygdala seems to be naturally programmed with some stimuli that will be perceived as a threat. Things such as fears of predators, angry facial expressions, snakes, insects, heights, etc. Some scientists believe this to be a sort of biological programming through evolution. If you look at children, they are naturally more afraid of heights or falling than of an airplane. This tells us that what the amygdala fears can be programmed to an extent. If we couldn't program or reprogram the biological fears built in us through evolution, it is doubtful that we could love sharp-toothed animals like cats or dogs and treat them as part of our families (Pittmann & Karle, 2015).

Furthermore, there are so many things and scenarios the amygdala doesn't naturally fear. Like we've mentioned before: we learn to fear through past life experiences. Our little almond in the limbic system keeps learning what to fear as we go through experiences.

So with all this in mind, it might be difficult to know when you are having an anxiety or panic attack, or just a learned reaction to fear.

Here are some common triggers for expected or unexpected anxiety attacks:

- High pressure, stressful jobs.
- Driving (especially in traffic).
- Social situations.
- Phobias (like claustrophobia; the fear of small places or acrophobia; the fear of heights).
- Caffeine.
- Thyroid issues.
- Withdrawal from drugs or alcohol.
- Memories of traumatic experiences.
- Chronic pain (to the extent of conditions like Fibromyalgia).
- Chronic illnesses like irritable bowel syndrome, asthma, heart disease, etc.

- Overexposure to ongoing stress and worries like work and debt.
- Going through a stressful life event like going through a divorce, or losing a loved one.
- Another mental health disorder like depression, PTSD, or OCD.

Now that you are more familiar with how the brain works with fearful triggers during an emergency response and how a panic attack manifests in the body, you should probably get that it could be a serious condition. If you frequently get panic attacks and keep you from living a joyful life, it might be good to get a proper diagnosis from a doctor to make sure you don't have any chemical imbalances or other mental disorders that might be underlying.,

ELEVEN

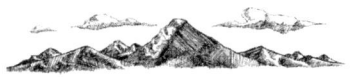

Exercises

Abdominal Breathing

Pretty much every wellness coach or expert will tell you that intentional breathing has excellent advantages for your health in general. However, we have already determined that people suffering from anxiety have a great struggle in staying present. This is because their mind is running loose between the past and/or the future. Breathing is a great tool to assist in consciously pulling yourself back into the present. Your calm is just a few breaths away.

Though breathing alone isn't a one-stop-complete-fix for deep-seated anxieties, it does a great job at soothing and easing anxiety and your garden-variety stresses. However, we need to consciously rethink how we breathe.

Why We've Become a Society of Chest-Breathers

Well, science tells us that the average person takes around 23,000 breaths per day. Our bodies are such amazing hosts that have a natural intelligence running these automated processes that keep us alive. Basically, this intelligence is like background apps running on your smart devices: checking that all central systems are running smoothly. If some sort of malfunction is picked up, a notification pops up on your device, guiding you through the steps to assist with a fix.

If you become aware that you actually have "built-in-apps" running in your body, it's quite easy to look out for the "pop-up," indicating a malfunction or something malicious in your system. When you are experiencing any of the symptoms of anxiety in your body, you could see them as a "pop-up" from your natural intelligence system running in the background. One of the possible fixes to get the system running smoothly again is breathing.

Naturally, we tend to be chest-breathers, especially when we experience some form of stress. When we're exposed to a threat, our fight, flight, or freeze (FFF-responses) responses kick in, which applies to our breathing response. We start breathing at a Speedy-Gonzalez-pace to get ample oxygen to our muscles and our heart so our bodies can flee or fight. Alternatively, we freeze and stop breathing altogether for a moment and feel overwhelmed and weak.

But like we mentioned earlier, we don't have predators that hunt us down anymore. Our fear and stresses now come from information overload, personal confrontations, traffic, etc. We're enveloped in these stresses daily. Because our FFF-responses are temporary and are ebbing and flowing into our lives, we've become accustomed to being in a state of tension. Believe it or not, our FFF-responses never completely shut down. They keep running in the background parallel to our natural intelligence that is scanning for malware. The result is that we tend to become shallow chest-breathers, and we tend to only do the minimum "fix" to stay alive.

Why We Should Become Belly-Breathers

Breathing from your abdominals stimulates the vagus nerve. But "what-the-vague-is-your-vagus-nerve" anyway?

The vagus nerve stretches from the head down the neck,

through the chest right down into the colon. When this nerve is stimulated, it activates your body's relaxation response, which reduces your heart rate and lowers your blood pressure —this aids in lowering your stress levels.

But how do you guide your natural intelligence closer to belly-breathing and away from the tendency to "quick-fix" with chest-breathing? Well, here are some simple exercises:

Exercise 1: "Chairing" is caring.

- Sit comfortably in a chair while leaning forward.
- Place your elbows on your knees.
- Breathe naturally in this position.

This chair position forces you to breathe from your abdominals, so it's an excellent way to experience belly-breathing if you're not familiar with it.

Exercise 2: Exhale longer than you inhale.

Breathing deeply is excellent, but we often take deep breaths to focus on breathing longer. Inhaling breaths are linked to our sympathetic nervous systems that control our FFF-responses. On the other hand, exhaling is linked to our parasympathetic nervous system that has an impact on our body's ability to relax. If you take too many deep breaths too fast, you can trigger your body into hyperventilation. This would not be conducive to calming your anxiety. Consequently, before taking in a deep breath, try counterintuitively exhaling instead. Push all of the air out of your lungs and let your lungs do the work of naturally inhaling fresh air.

Next, you can focus on taking more time to exhale. Count if you must: inhale for five seconds, exhale for seven seconds.

Repeat this exercise for two to five minutes. The great thing about this exercise is that you can do it in any comfortable position.

Exercise 3: Practice focusing on your breath.

When you are breathing deeply and focusing on a slow,

steady movement of in- and exhalation, you can reduce anxiety.

- Start by getting in a relaxed position and recognize how you generally are inhaling and exhaling. Search through your body with your mind.
- Take a slow deep breath in by way of the nose, while seeing how your belly and upper body is expanding.
- Practice a slow deep breath in through the nose, while seeing how your stomach and upper body is expanding.
- Exhale when you feel you need to and add a sigh if you wish. A sigh is a great way to release some tension.
- Repeat this for 2-5 minutes and concentrate on the rise and fall of your belly and upper body.
- Select a single word (calm, safe, worthy, loved, etc.) to now focus on when you exhale.
- When you inhale, envision the fresh air washing over you like a wave.
- Use that powerful imagination we spoke about in chapter 5 to see how each breath you breathe out is carrying negative energies and thoughts away from you.
- If you get distracted - just gently bring your focus back to your breathing.

How frequently do I need to practice belly-breathing?

Once every hour is a good ratio. Try programming a reminder on your phone or smartwatch to make you get into a habit.

Alternatively, 10 – 15 times throughout the day is a good option.

The more you practice belly-breathing, the quicker it will become a habit that your body naturally engages in – especially when you find yourself in a stressful situation.

Yoga

Before we just jump into yoga exercises, I want you to understand the profound connection between yoga and how it can be seen as a tremendous cognitive behavioral therapy-based strategy to keep a firm grip on your anxiety.

A brief introduction to the Ashtanga 8-limbed path of yoga.

The Ashtanga 8-limbed path of yoga has been historically used by yoga teachers as a guiding path to enlightenment. If we were to link this path to the management of anxiety, one could basically call it a treatment plan for anxiety through yoga.

Without getting too technical on the Sanskrit, we're going to have a quick look at how the path looks if we apply it to the management of our anxiety.

The first two steps in the Ashtanga path refer to the Yamas and Niyamas. These are behaviors that yogis cultivate to improve their quality of life. Examples of these behaviors include nonviolence, contentment, moderation, and perseverance.

The third step to enlightenment is the Asanas, which refer to the actual yoga poses that most of us know, like the downward dog, child pose, etc.

After the poses, Pranayama is practiced. This is breath control to change how we breathe, to deeper and more conscious belly-breathing (sound familiar?).

Then you get to Pratyahara, which focuses on drawing the senses inward and shutting out external stimuli to get in touch with what we are feeling, thinking, and doing.

As each step in this path prepares you for the next level.

One now moves into Dharana or concentration. Once all senses have been drawn inward, one can now focus. It doesn't matter so much what the focus is on, as long as one learns how to focus on one thing or aspect.

From this point, one reaches Dhyana or meditation. Concentration and meditation may seem more or less the same, but to be in a meditative state is where one is aware, without focus. Once you are in this state of consciousness, you can explore what you are thinking, feeling, and doing from a place of non-judgment and non-attachment.

After you have worked through all these steps, one hopes to reach Ashtanga's final state, Samadhi, or bliss. Here we feel totally integrated with ourselves and possibly our higher power or just a part of the greater community.

Now with this, all in mind, doesn't yoga seem like a one-stop exercise that incorporates most of the skills we have been introducing throughout the book?

Enough theory, let's have a look at a few poses that are great to alleviate anxiety.

Hero Pose

1. Place yourself in a kneeling posture with your knees placed together, and your feet spread a little wider than your hips.
2. Make sure the tops of your feet remain flat on the floor.
3. If you experience some discomfort, try using a cushion or block under your buttocks, thighs, or calves.
4. Put your hands on your thighs.
5. Make sure you sit in an upright posture where you open your chest and elongate your spine.
6. Hold for up to 5 minutes and relax.

Standing Forward Bend

1. Place your feet more or less hip-width apart and place your hands on your hips.
2. Hinge at your hips into a forward fold while exhaling. Make sure to keep a slight bend in your knees.
3. Let your hands comfortably rest on the floor. If you can't reach the floor yet, use a block or step to help you.
4. Tuck your chin within your chest while you maintain the pose.
5. You want the tension in your lower back and hips to be released. If you are not experiencing this, slightly adjust your body until you feel the desired effect. It helps if your head and neck hang heavy toward the floor.
6. Hold for 1-3 minutes.

Fish Pose

1. While you are seated, stretch your legs out in front of you.
2. Hands should be positioned underneath your buttocks with your palms facing towards the ground.
3. Then expand your chest and squeeze your elbows towards each other behind you.
4. After that, gently lean back and move into a position of resting on your forearms and elbows. Keep your chest lifted during this move by pressing into your arms.
5. Should you experience discomfort, let your head hang back toward the floor or rest it on something like a cushion, folded towel, or yoga block.

6. Maintain this pose for up to 1 minute.

Child's Pose

1. Sink back into your heels from a kneeling position.
2. Move your hands forward as if they are walking towards something.
3. Then, let your torso lean heavy into your thighs, with your forehead resting on the floor.
4. You can choose to rest your arms next to your body or stretch them out in front of you.
5. Hold this pose for 3-5 minutes and relax.

Head-to-Knee Forward Bend

1. With your left leg extended, sit on the edge of a cushion, block, or folded towel.
2. Take the sole of your right foot and press it into your left thigh.
3. If you feel that you need some extra support, you can place a block or cushion under one or both knees.
4. Inhale while stretching your arms forward and over your head.
5. Exhale while you hinge at the hips, and stretch your spine into a forward fold.
6. Rest your hands anywhere comfortable - your body or the floor will do!
7. Hold this pose for 2-3 minutes.
8. Repeat on the other side.

Legs up the Wall Pose

1. Place your yoga mat near a wall that can help you stretch your legs and support you.

2. Then position your bum as close to the wall as possible. Get intimate with the wall. It helps if you lay curled up on your side first, with your hip against the wall, and then turn over gently onto your back when you reach the position where you can stretch your legs up straight against the wall.
3. Your arms should be relaxed next to your sides with your palms facing up.
4. Close your eyes and focus on your breath. It's great to consider a sleeping mask if you tend to get distracted.
5. In this position, you take deep breaths. Inhale for 5 counts, exhale for five counts. Feel tension being relieved from your whole body. This is a great position to try if you want to slow your heart rate down fast. This position you can hold as long as you like or find comfortable.

Seated Forward Bend

1. With your legs stretched right in front of you, sit up straight on your mat. Gently move your seated weight from one side of your body to the other, so you feel almost pressed, or stuck into the ground.
2. Reach your arms up, lengthen your spine, and then reach for your toes with your heart.
3. Go as far as your body can. You want to feel a stretch but no pain.
4. Keep your back flat if you can because this will target the stretch in your hamstrings. If you round your back, this stretch will reach your back muscles more. Both are effective, and you can choose what works best for you.
5. Toes can be toes pointed forward or flexed upwards. Attempt both and see what you prefer.

6. Hold 2-5 minutes and slowly roll-up.

Cat/Cow Pose

1. Position yourself on all fours. Make sure your hands are beneath your shoulders and your knees below your hip bones. Your back must remain in a straight, neutral position at the start.
2. Lower your belly, pull your shoulder blades towards each other, open your chest and lift your gaze upward into cow pose. Do this while inhaling.
3. Pull your navel in, gaze down toward it, draw your shoulder blades apart, and exhale it into cat pose.
4. Repeat these moves focusing on how your breath partners with each movement.
5. Progress slowly to feel the shift of each vertebra of your spine.
6. Use this pose to exercise conscious breathing - not just as a relaxing stretch!
7. Keep at it for at least 5 minutes, if possible.

Corpse Pose

Don't let this pose fool you! Physically it doesn't require much effort, but it can be challenging for the mind to master.

1. Lie on your back on your mat. With your palms facing up, your arms should be by your sides, and your legs should be completely relaxed.
2. If your lower back is experiencing tension, support it by putting a pillow or block under your knees.
3. Close your eyes, and take your concentration though your face, letting every facial muscle know that it should relax.
4. Practice in and out deep breathing until you feel

very relaxed. Do not let your mind wander beyond your breath.
5. Hold this pose for up to 5 minutes.

It is my genuine hope for you that these poses will become part of your nature. When the world seems overwhelming, may you return to these and connect your body and your mind with these poses and so, also soothe your soul.

Don't forget to consciously clear your mind through deep breathing (remember how we visualized breathing out toxic, negative energies earlier?). May yoga be an excellent omen and reminder that anxiety won't last forever and that you do have everything you need, right inside of you, to create a safe, calm, and relaxed space.

TWELVE

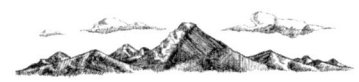

Thought Versus Reality

WE'VE DETERMINED THAT ANXIETY IS A PURE EMOTION. THE way it is experienced, how we interact with, and react to it can be everything but simple.

Now on the spectrum of anxiety, an important thing to note is that anxiety can morph into an experience that can distort your reality. Anxiety basically has the power to change the way our mind processes information. It can literally make us experience all of the symptoms of fear even when there isn't fear in sight.

Remember the example of the piece of bark that was perceived as a scorpion?

When a person or situation denies you your reality, you are actually allowed to learn to really trust yourself. When you choose to honor your own reality, you position yourself to begin healing your anxious nature without the validation of others.

Unfortunately, for some, it's not as simple as I last mentioned. For some anxiety sufferers, their anxiety can be so severe that it feels like they are losing touch with the world. People with anxiety often don't even know that it is their anxiety that is causing their warped world view.

So how does one know if you are experiencing a distorted reality? Look out for these signs:

- You feel like something's off, but you are unable to picture or verbalize what's wrong.
- You often find yourself lost and confused or related feelings to loss and confusion.
- You feel like your brain simply stops processing the information around you like you're going into your own bubble.
- You frequently feel like you are looking at yourself from outside your body.

When you find that your anxiety is causing such an immense impact on your life that you struggle to form coherent thoughts, you might be experiencing 'derealization.' This is the type of defense and coping mechanism that the brain puts into play when extreme anxiety levels are present.

Derealization is often present during panic attacks or even in situations of intense stress. This kind of reality distortion is unique to each individual. The cause isn't precisely precise, but it seems to be how the mind shuts down certain elements when extreme stress is present because the effect of the stress could potentially damage the brain. So it's almost like the brain is taking a "time-out" from the world. However, when this happens, the person who is suffering from that level of anxiety and derealization is left feeling very out of sorts.

This "off" feeling of derealization can construct some anxieties of its own and just make the poor anxiety sufferer feel even more disconnected - sometimes to the extent that they think their minds are turning to schizophrenic tendencies. If this kind of paranoia and downright weird feeling is prolonged, they might even feel that they have a brain tumor and start monitoring themselves in a horrible thinking pattern that just deepens their anxiety. This is a very unfortunate reality for many people and a reality that doesn't have a quick or easy fix.

Firstly, there really are mental disorders and other health conditions that can cause a total loss of touch with reality. If you have a genuine concern about your level of connection with reality, go seek help from a professional. Here's the fact that you are conscious enough to think that you are losing touch with reality should be enough reassurance that you are still fine.

People who have altogether lost touch with reality and live in a warped reality have no clue that their reality is warped or distorted. It's essential to recognize that becoming lost in your thoughts due to anxiety is not actually that dangerous. It's also not a permanent state of being. A distorted reality from anxiety rarely surfaces at any other point than during an anxiety or panic attack.

If you do feel that your reality is distorted, here are a few things you can try to pull yourself back into reality. Many therapists simply recommend doing something that requires you to be present and then focusing on the sensations generated through the activity. Examples include:

- Running your hands under cold water and concentrating on the feeling cold water is creating on your hands.
- Literally pinching yourself to remind you that you are real.
- Jumping up and down or some form of quick cardio movement to get the blood pumping.
- Focus on one specific color in your surroundings. Then start counting other objects in your environment with the same color.

Even though this may sound silly, these activities pull you towards being present. The only sure way to prevent a loss of reality from returning to your thoughts is to make sure that you manage your anxiety levels. Never allow your levels to reach such an extreme point. In other words, just use what you've learned throughout this book!

THIRTEEN

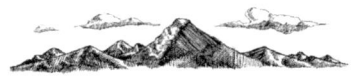

Getting Unstuck From a Thought

WHEN WE ARE WORKING ON HEALING AND BALANCING OUR anxiety, we're not treating a mental illness. We identify unresolved trauma, get to know our responses to specific triggers, and navigate our coping mechanisms to aid in well-being rather than destructive behaviors. We are rewiring your subconscious programming.

When I get stuck in thoughts, I can reflect on the fact that I can experience two truths. The reality I created in my mind due to my subconscious programming, versus the present situation I find myself in.

A great way of getting unstuck from a thought is to get your body unstuck and moving. Think about the "Let's Do It" technique I explained earlier. When you start engaging in an action, it pulls your thought towards the activity you are participating in.

The Wiggle Strategy

When you are stuck in thought, your body might also be tensed up and stuck. A simple technique to get your mind back into your body is simply to take a stand. Then you wiggle, wiggle, wiggle - don't mind the jiggly bits. Through wiggling, you might also trigger some childlike feelings that can generate a little laughter. Sometimes tension melts away through a hint of silliness.

The Jumping Jack Flash Strategy

No, it's not just an amazing Rolling Stones song. Getting some jumping jacks on in a flash can be a tremendous counterintuitive strategy to get you out of your mind. We've already gone through some breathing techniques, which is fabulous. But doing a few jumping jacks can be a great way to guide your thoughts and physical responses away from panic attacks. If you are so stuck in your mind, you might find that meditation and deep belly breathing can actually deepen your feelings of anxiety in some instances. Thus if you get into some jumping jacks, you will still be regulating your breathing. Instead of trying to slow the energy level of your anxiety down, you will be working up your own energy level to match the pace. You won't only do some rewiring of your anxious feelings and regulate the physical symptoms of anxiety-like shallow breathing. Still, you will also be burning some calories from the emotional eating binge earlier. See, it's a win-win!

The Angry Screamer Strategy

Most often, anger is positioned as a negative emotion. However, if all of the anxiety in your mind is weighing you down and causing frustration, it might not be such a bad plan to let go of some of that frustration. If you've been clinging to some negative emotions that you haven't expressed, grabbing a pillow or getting outside and just yelling out loud in anger and frustration can do wonders for releasing some of the negative energy you've been carrying around in your thoughts. You also don't really have to yell like a maniac (though it works great for myself), but you can phone a friend and just vent. The point is to express your anger and frustration and to not let it pile up and cause an ample space in your mind.

So basically, to get mentally unstuck, you should physically let loose!

FOURTEEN

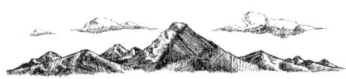

The Road Ahead

GOING FORWARD, I BELIEVE IT'S TIME WE NEED TO MAKE PEACE with the fact that our lives will always have some level of uncertainty involved. Ironically, the only thing in life that is certain is probably uncertainty.

Essentially, there is no way of altogether avoiding anxiety because anxiety is a worry about a future issue, for which we have no specific answer. What we can do is:

- Take a moment to evaluate the actual risks that are surrounding you.
- Then work on maximizing how prepared you are to face danger or uncertainty. If you feel ready to face danger, you're communicating to your amygdala that you are prepared to face whatever comes your way - no need for an overreaction.
- When trauma hits, make sure you deal with it.
- Make a conscious effort to laugh and play.
- Allow yourself to be vulnerable and honest about your anxiety to the people around you. You'll be surprised how many people are aching to share their vulnerabilities, too, but are afraid. Be brave

and take the first step. Remember, anxiety is a shared human emotion. We need to help and support each other to make this world a gentler, kinder place to live in.

The road ahead for you is filled with new discoveries and healing.

Building Your Support Network

Timon had Pumba, and Pumba had Timon. Together they had support. You do not have to deal with your anxiety relapses alone.

Talk to your friends and family about your emotional distress. If they are your point of emotional distress, grab your smartphone, hop onto Google, and search for your nearest support group. You've got this, and you're definitely not alone. Likewise, don't be reluctant to shop around for a group that goes with your vibe.

Don't underestimate the connections you can make through joining a yoga class and not just doing some of the stretches mentioned in Chapter 6 or hopping on to YouTube. Chances are you'll meet some very like-minded folks in class!

You also don't just have to stick to anxiety support groups or yoga. When we reach the chapter on how to not worry what other people think and how to grapple with the fear of failure, we touched on the importance of getting to know yourself, your values, and what you like. If you like being creative, then go to a pottery class. Make a friend who is also creative. If someone is supporting a part of you that makes you happier, that's great too. Sometimes we seek support groups and help when we require damage control, when, in fact, support should actually assist in maintaining a healthy balance in your life.

Don't get too serious about getting a support network into

place - make it fun. Hold the individuals who feel like sunshine close. Feed your conscious cortex with reassuring messages of calm, contentment and worthiness, so that little amygdala won't have to feel programmed to jump in and overreact in a situation that's not that bad at all. And allow yourself to be deeply seen - anxiety and all! Remember, you are not anxiety. You have anxiety in you. Also, you are not the only one confronting anxiety. We're all in this together.

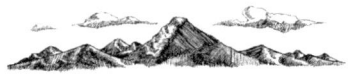

Conclusion

Congrats, Hakuna Matata-er! You made it through. It is my heartfelt desire that you feel absolutely empowered by your new insights into anxiety.

Remember that even though life will never really have "no worries for the rest of your days," you have the power to at least live by your own "problem-free, philosophy."

You can choose to see problems as opportunities. You can choose to breathe from your belly and not your chest. You can choose to say "Let's Do It" instead of getting lost in procrastinating thoughts. You can choose to grip your anxiety with both hands and embrace it for all the things you will learn. Of course, you can hop on over to your favorite retailer and give us a Hakuna Matata rating if this book has moved you forward.

References

American Psychological Association. (n.d). Anxiety. Retrieved May 2, 2020 from: https://www.apa.org/topics/anxiety/

Ami, T. (n.d.). 6 Yoga poses that help alleviate anxiety. Retrieved May 11, 2020 from: https://www.doyou.com/6-yoga-poses-that-help-alleviate-anxiety-38992/

Allers, R. & Minkoff, R. (Directors). (1994). The Lion King [Film]. Walt Disney Feature Animation.

Azarian, B. (2016, September 6). How anxiety warps your perception. Retrieved May 3, 2020 from: https://www.bbc.com/future/article/20160928-how-anxiety-warps-your-perception

Brené, B. (2019). List of core emotions [PDF File]. Retrieved from: https://brenebrown.com/wp-content/uploads/2019/06/List-of-Core-Emotions-1-2020.pdf

Cronkleton, E. (2018, June 6). Yoga for anxiety: 11 Poses to Try. Retrieved May 11, 2020 from: https://www.doyou.com/6-yoga-poses-that-help-alleviate-anxiety-38992/

Elliot, CH. & Smith LL. (2010). Overcoming anxiety for dummies [PDF File] 2nd ed.). Wiley Publishing, Inc. Retrieved from: https://www.pdfdrive.com/overcoming-anxiety-for-dummies-2nd-edition-e19451769.html

References

Felman, A. (2020, January 11). What to know about anxiety. Retrieved May 2, 2020 from: https://www.medicalnewstoday.com/articles/323454

Kipman, S. (2019, June 18). 15 Highly successful people who failed on their way to success. Retrieved 8 May, 2020 from: https://www.lifehack.org/articles/productivity/15-highly-successful-people-who-failed-their-way-success.html

Marques, L. (2018, July 18). Do I have anxiety or worry: What's the difference?. Retrieved May 3, 2020 from: https://www.health.harvard.edu/blog/ease-anxiety-and-stress-take-a-belly-breather-2019042616521

Merriam-Webster. (n.d.) Anxiety. In Merriam-Webster.com dictionary. Retrieved May 2, 2020 from: https://www.merriam-webster.com/dictionary/anxiety

Pittman, CM. & Karle, E.M. (2015). Rewire your anxious brain: How to use the neuroscience of fear to end anxiety, panic & worry [PDF File]. New Harbinger Publications, Inc. Retrieved from: https://www.pdfdrive.com/rewire-your-anxious-brain-how-to-use-the-neuroscience-of-fear-to-end-anxiety-panic-and-worry-e157833544.html

Sack, D. (2016, October 17). 8 Ways to stop worrying about what other people think. Retrieved May 8, 2020 from: https://www.psychologytoday.com/za/blog/where-science-meets-the-steps/201610/8-ways-stop-worrying-about-what-other-people-think

Shaikh, F. (2018, October 27). How anxiety can cause distorted reality. Retrieved May 4, 2020 from: https://www.calmclinic.com/anxiety/symptoms/distorted-reality

Solan, M. (2019, April 26). Ease anxiety and stress: Take a (belly) breather. Retrieved May 3, 2020 from: https://www.health.harvard.edu/blog/ease-anxiety-and-stress-take-a-belly-breather-2019042616521

Wilson, R. (n.d.). Help for anxiety, panic, phobias and OCD. Retrieved May 5, 2020 from: https://www.anxieties.com/1/free

References

Winston, SM. & Seif MN. (2017). Overcoming Unwanted Intrusive Thoughts: A CBT-based guide to getting over frightening, obsessive, or disturbing thoughts [PDF File]. New Harbinger Publications, Inc. Retrieved from: https://www.pdfdrive.com/overcoming-unwanted-intrusive-thoughts-a-cbt-based-guide-to-getting-over-frightening-obsessive-or-disturbing-thoughts-e176334635.html

BBC WorldWide Service. (2016, August 22). What is the best way to deal with anxiety [Audio Podcast]. Retrieved from: https://podcasts.apple.com/za/podcast/the-forum/id284278990?i=1000374410170

About the Author

Monique Joiner Siedlak is a writer, witch, and warrior on a mission to awaken people to their greatest potential through the power of storytelling infused with mysticism, modern paganism, and new age spirituality. At the young age of 12, she began rigorously studying the fascinating philosophy of Wicca. By the time she was 20, she was self-initiated into the craft, and hasn't looked back ever since. To this day, she has authored over 40 books pertaining to the magick and mysteries of life.

To find out more about Monique Joiner Siedlak artistically, spiritually, and personally, feel free to visit her **official website**.

www.mojosiedlak.com

- facebook.com/mojosiedlak
- twitter.com/mojosiedlak
- instagram.com/mojosiedlak
- pinterest.com/mojosiedlak
- bookbub.com/authors/monique-joiner-siedlak

More Books by Monique Joiner Siedlak

Practical Magick
  Wiccan Basics
  Candle Magick
  Wiccan Spells
  Love Spells
  Abundance Spells
  Herb Magick
  Moon Magick
  Creating Your Own Spells
  Gypsy Magic
  Protection Magick
  Celtic Magick
  Shamanic Magick

African Magic
  Hoodoo
  Seven African Powers: The Orishas
  Cooking for the Orishas
  Lucumi: The Ways of Santeria
  Voodoo of Louisiana
  Haitian Vodou

Orishas of Trinidad
Connecting with your Ancestors

The Yoga Collective
Yoga for Beginners
Yoga for Stress
Yoga for Back Pain
Yoga for Weight Loss
Yoga for Flexibility
Yoga for Advanced Beginners
Yoga for Fitness
Yoga for Runners
Yoga for Energy
Yoga for Your Sex Life
Yoga To Beat Depression and Anxiety
Yoga for Menstruation
Yoga to Detox Your Body
Yoga to Tone Your Body

A Natural Beautiful You
Creating Your Own Body Butter
Creating Your Own Body Scrub
Creating Your Own Body Spray

Thank you for reading my book.
I really appreciate all your feedback and would love to hear what you have to say! Please leave your review at your favorite retailer!

www.ingramcontent.com/pod-product-compliance
Lightning Source LLC
Chambersburg PA
CBHW071305040426
42444CB00009B/1874